Understanding

ALLERGIES

Dr Joanne Clough

D0773821

Published by Family Doctor Publications Limited
in association with the British Medical Association

IMPORTANT NOTICE

Family Doctor Publications, PO Box 4664, Poole, Dorset BH15 1NN

Medical Editor: Dr Tony Smith
Consultant Editor: Mary Fox
Cover Artist: Dave Eastbury
Medical Artist: Peter Cox Associates
Design: MPG Design, Blandford Forum, Dorset
Printing: Nuffield Press, Abingdon, Oxon, using acid-free paper

ISBN: 1 903474 08 6

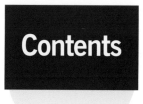

Contents

Introduction

An allergy is a damaging response of the immune system to a substance that is normally harmless. The number of people affected in the United Kingdom has increased dramatically since the early 1970s and it continues to rise. As many as one in three people in the UK now suffer from a medical problem caused by or associated with allergy. It is predicted that a similar increase will be seen in the developing countries as they become more Westernised.

This is because many of the factors thought to be responsible for the increase are related to the Western lifestyle. These factors include our unnaturally refined diet, the early introduction of certain foods to the infant diet, our style of housing, the popularity of indoor furry pets, our increased exposure to chemicals that may cause allergies, households made up of smaller numbers of people and our exposure to tobacco smoke. Many of these factors seem to be especially potent in small children.

The most common diseases in which allergy plays a part are asthma, hay fever (also called allergic rhinitis), allergies affecting the skin (including eczema and contact dermatitis) and food allergy.

Asthma causes episodes of wheezing, coughing and shortness of breath that can be triggered by a range of things, including the common cold, exercise, contact with furry animals, a high pollen count and exposure to tobacco smoke. It is a frequent problem in children, affecting as many as one in every seven school-aged children. Asthma is slightly less common in adults – affecting about one in ten – but is still a major cause of ill-health. Many studies have confirmed that asthma is becoming more common, but little is known about why.

Hay fever can be a seasonal

condition, causing symptoms in late spring and summer, or may cause problems all year round. Its symptoms may not sound serious – a running or blocked nose, watery itchy eyes and sneezing – but they make the lives of hay fever sufferers a misery, and may interfere with work, study and sleep. The exact number of people with hay fever is difficult to judge but it is thought that as many as 20 per cent of the British population have hay fever at some stage in their lives.

Skin allergies may take several different forms. Probably the best known is eczema, but other problems such as contact dermatitis, urticaria (hives) and facial swelling (angio-oedema) may also be the result of allergy. Although skin allergy can affect both sexes, more and more women in particular are developing new allergies. This may be because the average woman uses five different cosmetic and skin care products on her skin every day, and these are likely to contain around 100 different chemicals, any one of which could cause an allergic reaction.

Although almost a fifth of people in the UK think that they are allergic to at least one food, the actual figure is much lower – allergy is often incorrectly blamed for causing symptoms that are not truly allergic in nature. Only about two per cent have a true food allergy.

However, there are a number of other reasons why a food might disagree with you. A food may have caused an upset once, so the person assumes that it will always cause a problem and the term 'allergy' is used, incorrectly, to describe what happened. A person may develop unpleasant associations with a particular food (correctly called food aversion) and think that he or she is allergic to it – even if he or she has either no symptoms at all or only a minor upset when the food is included in the diet.

The problem of misdiagnosis is not confined to food allergy. Allergy seems to have become fashionable, particularly among young women. In addition, some alternative practitioners use tests that have not been scientifically assessed and these tests may misdiagnose allergy. The careful and accurate diagnosis of allergic problems is important for two reasons. First, sufferers may be making major changes in their diet or in their lifestyle – in the belief that they have an allergic disease – and, if they do not, these changes may interfere with the quality of their lives for no good reason. Second, labelling their problem incorrectly prevents them from discovering the true reason for their problem and finding the best treatment for it.

This book explains what happens in the body when an

allergy occurs and how to decide whether or not allergy is the problem. It also describes the different ways of diagnosing allergy and discusses the different treatments available. Finally, useful information about living with allergies is given.

If you have an allergy-related problem this book should help you to find your way through the allergy maze. No book can be a substitute for consultation with a doctor, but by making you better informed and well prepared, this book will help you to be more in control of your allergic problems and to manage them better.

KEY POINTS

✓ One in three people in the UK are affected by allergy

✓ Allergy is often misdiagnosed

What is allergy?

Humans have a sophisticated defence system that has evolved to protect us against a range of threats, including micro-organisms (such as bacteria, viruses and parasites), chemical substances and even cancer. This defence system, the immune system, is made up of a large number of different cell types and special proteins. These work together in a complex way to enable us to distinguish our own cells ('self') from harmful cells ('non-self') and so to destroy abnormal or invading cells. However, occasionally the immune system reacts to substances that are harmless, and the resulting allergic reaction causes damage to the surrounding tissues.

An allergic reaction is an overreaction of the immune defence system, in which it responds inappropriately to a normally harmless environmental substance, causing troublesome or even life-threatening effects. The term 'allergy' is sometimes used to describe just about any kind of illness. In this book, the term will be used much more precisely to mean a heightened or exaggerated response of the immune system to a substance that is normally harmless.

The different parts of the immune system include the white blood cells, the spleen, the lymph nodes, the thymus gland, and the many small glands within the lining of the respiratory and intestinal tracts. There are several different types of white blood cell, including lymphocytes, neutrophils, eosinophils, mast cells and macrophages. All of these are controlled by protein messengers (hormones), which are produced by the white blood cells.

IN THE HEALTHY PERSON

The prime purpose of the immune system is to protect us from micro-organisms that might otherwise kill us. When one of these, such as the measles virus or the bacterium *Staphylococcus aureus*, attacks the body for the first time, cells within the lymph nodes, lungs or bowel recognise it as foreign (non-self) because of certain protein molecules (known as antigens) on its surface, and bring it to the attention of the lymphocytes. One type of lymphocyte (T lymphocyte) produces protein messengers that stimulate other cells (the B lymphocytes) to produce purpose-built proteins called antibodies. These antibodies are specifically made to fit with and bind on to the antigens on the invading cell's surface. Once there, they send signals to teams of killer cells, which move in and kill the invader. Each time a different antigen is met, antibodies are made specifically against it, and the body can make millions of different ones.

The process of recognising an antigen and making antibodies against it for the first time is called sensitisation. It may take a few days for the body's response to reach full strength. However, for the rest of your life your immune system is able to remember harmful micro-organisms and, if the same organism attacks again, it is immediately recognised. No other organ of the body (apart from the brain) has the property of memory.

If the same micro-organism strikes again, as soon as its antigens are recognised, the T lymphocytes send chemical messages to the group of B lymphocytes that have a specific memory for the invader, and these multiply very quickly and produce large amounts of antibody, which helps to kill the harmful cells. Other white cells produce chemicals such as histamine and leukotrienes, which increase the blood supply to the area involved and make the blood vessels more leaky. This allows other white blood cell types, such as the macrophage, which are able to eat and destroy the invading cells, to reach the area. We can see evidence of this process when a skin wound becomes infected. The area becomes red and swollen because of the increased blood supply, and may be hot and sore as a result of certain chemicals produced in the course of the immune reaction. This process is known as inflammation.

IN THE ALLERGIC PERSON

If you develop an allergy it is because, even though your immune system works perfectly well against the antigens associated with viruses, bacteria and parasites, it also reacts to other antigens that should be completely harmless.

HOW THE IMMUNE SYSTEM DEALS WITH HARMFUL CELLS

The immune (defence) system is made up of many different cell types that work together to enable the body to distinguish between its own cells ('self') and harmful cells ('non-self'). The following sequence of five illustrations is a representation of how the immune system works to destroy invading micro-organisms.

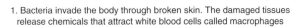

Broken skin

Invading bacterium

Blood vessel

1. Bacteria invade the body through broken skin. The damaged tissues release chemicals that attract white blood cells called macrophages

Macrophages destroying invading cells

Porous blood vessel

2. The chemicals also cause the underlying blood vessels to dilate, increasing the blood supply to the area and making the vessels more leaky, which causes the characteristics of inflammation and also allows macrophages to reach the invading cells

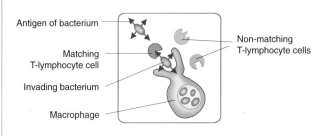

Antigen of bacterium

Non-matching T-lymphocyte cells

Matching T-lymphocyte cell

Invading bacterium

Macrophage

3. Some of the invading cells are destroyed by macrophages. Matching T-lymphocyte cells send signals to B-lymphocyte cells to make specific antibodies to deal with the invader

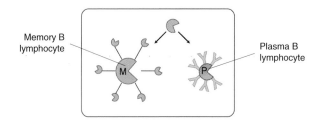

Memory B lymphocyte

Plasma B lymphocyte

4. The matching T-lymphocyte cell stimulates the production of two types of B lymphocyte: plasma cells which produce antibodies for immediate use and memory cells which are stored for future use

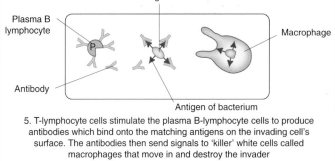

Invading bacterium

Plasma B lymphocyte

Macrophage

Antibody

Antigen of bacterium

5. T-lymphocyte cells stimulate the plasma B-lymphocyte cells to produce antibodies which bind onto the matching antigens on the invading cell's surface. The antibodies then send signals to 'killer' white cells called macrophages that move in and destroy the invader

These antigens are known as allergens. These are incorrectly seen as being dangerous by your immune system, which mounts an immune response against them. This response is called an allergic reaction, and you will have developed an allergy.

There are two stages in the development of an allergy, and the first is sensitisation (see page 5 and box on page 6). This process happens when an allergen is encountered by the immune system and antibodies are made against it, despite it being harmless. These antibodies are of the same type as those that protect us against parasites such as worms, flukes and amoebae, and are known as immunoglobulin E or IgE for short – immunoglobulin is another name for an antibody. Parasites are much larger than other micro-organisms such as viruses and bacteria, and the body has had to find alternative ways of getting rid of them. IgE is different from other types of antibody in that it can attach itself to mast cells and basophils. These white blood cells contain thousands of toxic granules capable of killing parasites, which are released when an allergen binds to IgE on the cell surface.

After sensitisation, the immune system retains a memory of the allergen and will recognise it if it meets it again. Sensitisation does not produce any symptoms and you will not be aware that it is happening. You do not always become sensitised the first time that your body meets a particular allergen – a substance may be tolerated for many years before an allergy develops.

Once you have been sensitised, even a tiny quantity of that allergen can lead to an allergic reaction. The allergen binds to the IgE present on the surface of the mast cells and basophils, and the toxic granules are released. These contain potent irritant chemicals such as histamine and a number of different enzymes. If this reaction were the result of a parasitic infection, these chemicals would help to kill and digest the invading organisms. If, however, the immune system is reacting against a harmless allergen such as pollen, these substances serve no useful purpose, but instead cause an increase in the blood supply to the tissues, leakage of fluid from the small blood vessels and local irritation. The result is hotness, redness, itching and swelling in the affected area, and the production of excess watery secretions. In addition, the muscles of the airways in the lungs and the bowel may go into spasm, causing wheezing, shortness of breath, abdominal colic and diarrhoea. This process gives us the symptoms that we associate with allergy.

HOW AN ALLERGY DEVELOPS

There are two stages in the development of an allergy: first sensitisation which does not produce any symptoms and then the allergic reaction.

Sensitisation
Sensitisation occurs when your body meets an allergen, recognises it as foreign and your white blood cells make a memory of it.

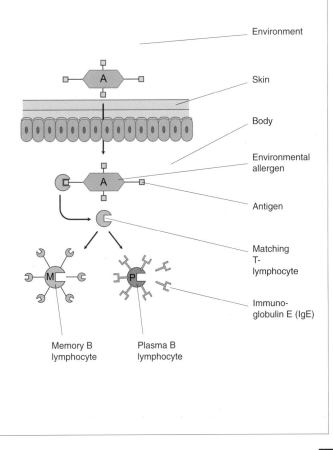

Environment

Skin

Body

Environmental allergen

Antigen

Matching T-lymphocyte

Immuno-globulin E (IgE)

Memory B lymphocyte

Plasma B lymphocyte

HOW AN ALLERGY DEVELOPS (contd)

Allergic reaction

1. Once the body is sensitised, if this allergen is met again, even a tiny amount can produce an allergic reaction.

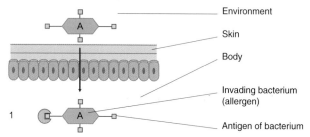

Environment

Skin

Body

Invading bacterium (allergen)

Antigen of bacterium

2. The allergen is recognised and this triggers the production of large quantities of the IgE antibody by the memory B lymphocytes.

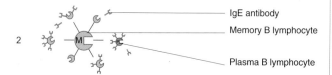

IgE antibody

Memory B lymphocyte

Plasma B lymphocyte

3. Some of the IgE antibody attaches to mast cells which contain toxic granules.

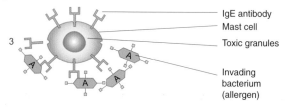

IgE antibody

Mast cell

Toxic granules

Invading bacterium (allergen)

4. The allergen causes the severe reaction as it binds to the IgE antibody present on the surface of the mast cell. The mast cell bursts releasing toxic chemicals which then cause the symptoms we associate with allergy.

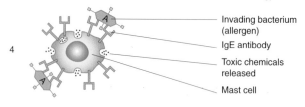

Invading bacterium (allergen)

IgE antibody

Toxic chemicals released

Mast cell

WHAT ARE THE MOST COMMON ALLERGENS?

Almost all allergens are made from proteins – organic compounds made of hydrogen, oxygen and nitrogen that are found in all living organisms. Occasionally, a non-protein substance can act as an allergen (for example, penicillin and other drugs), but only because they can attach themselves to a small protein molecule called a hapten inside the body. Virtually any protein can act as an allergen and new ones are being discovered all the time. The allergens most commonly causing allergies in the UK are described below.

House-dust mites

The house-dust mite is too small to be seen by the naked eye. It loves warm, humid conditions and large numbers can be found inside mattresses, bedding, pillows, soft furnishing and cuddly toys. House-dust mite allergy has become more common in recent times because double glazing, loft and wall insulation, and other energy-saving measures reduce ventilation inside our houses and encourage the warm, moist conditions that the house-dust mite needs.

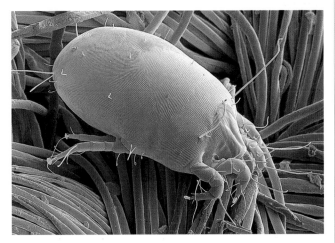

Electron micrograph of a house-dust mite.

The mite lives off scales of human skin which we constantly shed and which make up the majority of house dust. It is not the mites themselves but their faecal particles that act as allergens and cause allergies. These are so small that they can be suspended in the air for long periods of time and so can be inhaled though the nose and into the lungs, where they can cause the symptoms of hay fever and asthma. When they come into direct contact with the skin they can cause eczema. At least three-quarters of all allergy suffers in the UK are allergic to the house-dust mite.

Grass and tree pollen
Pollens are the male reproductive part of plants (or trees) that fertilise other plants of the same species. They are small grains and are carried either by insects or by air currents. The airborne pollens are very light and can be carried in the air for long periods of time. When these reach the eyes, nose or lungs of a sensitised person, they cause an allergic reaction commonly described as hay

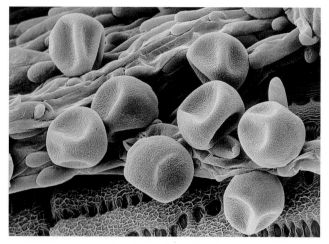

Electron micrograph of pollen grains.

fever. If breathed into the lungs they can make asthma worse.

Different plants produce their pollens at different times of the year and it is possible, using a pollen calendar, to work out which plants might be responsible for each individual's symptoms. The most common culprit is grass pollen, which is around from late April to early September.

Animal dander (skin scales and hair)

Most furry animals can cause an allergy. Allergens are in the skin scales, hairs and sometimes the saliva of animals. They can be spread widely throughout our homes, not just by animals but also on our clothing and shoes.

Seven of ten British households have a pet of some kind and pet allergens may cause about 40 per cent of all childhood asthma. Allergies to pets not only occur in their owners. The allergens are so potent and long lasting that they are easily spread – even non-pet owners can be exposed to enough allergen in their everyday life to become allergic.

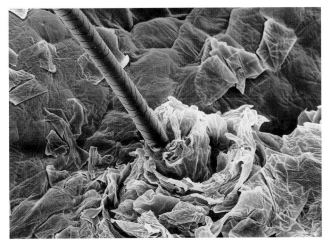

Electron micrograph of a human hair on the skin surface.

Food allergens
Many foods can act as allergens. The most common in children under the age of five are cows' milk and hen's eggs. Over the age of five years, other allergies are more common – such as to peanuts (which is not a true nut but a legume, that is, it grows as a seed in a pod like a pea), tree nuts, fish and shellfish.

Food allergies can take different forms, ranging from episodes of mild symptoms such as tingling and swelling of the lips to life-threatening attacks.

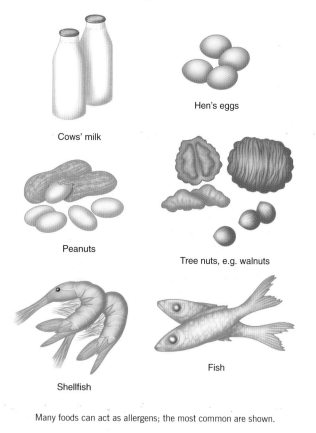

Cows' milk

Hen's eggs

Peanuts

Tree nuts, e.g. walnuts

Shellfish

Fish

Many foods can act as allergens; the most common are shown.

Moulds and spores

The spores from certain moulds and plants can trigger allergic reactions in some people, particularly in the autumn.

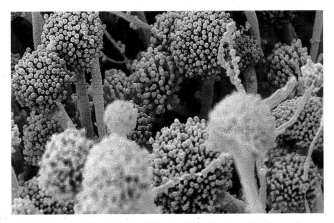

Electron micrograph of the fruiting bodies and spores of the fungus
Rhizopus oligosporus.

Drug allergies

Certain drugs, particularly some antibiotics, can cause allergic reactions. An allergy will never occur the first time a drug is administered but may do so on any subsequent occasion, even if the drug has been well tolerated in the past.

Insect stings

Although everyone finds insect stings unpleasant, in some people these can trigger allergic reactions that can be severe. Stings by bees and wasps are most commonly responsible.

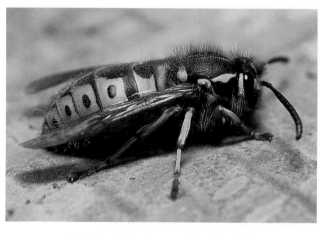

A common adult worker wasp – *Vespula vulgaris.*

Once you have developed an allergy, your body will always produce an allergic reaction whenever it meets this allergen again, even in minute amounts. However, the reaction will not necessarily be exactly the same each time. A number of things can affect the type and the extent of an allergic reaction. These include the amount of allergen involved, the part of your body exposed to the allergen, whether there are other factors present that enhance your allergic reaction (for example, a high level of air pollutants), and even how well you are at the time. In addition, the pattern of your allergic reactions may change as you get older. Some may become less pronounced with age, and it is even possible to 'grow out of' an allergy.

WHO DEVELOPS ALLERGIES?

Although we do not completely understand why it is that some people develop allergies and others do not, it is clear that allergies have a tendency to run in families. This inherited tendency towards allergy is called atopy.

In the near future it is likely that the genes (a gene is a small part of our genetic code made of DNA) responsible for atopy will be identified.

Atopic people produce excess quantities of the allergy antibody (IgE) when they come into contact with substances in their environment that can act as allergens.

Although atopy is inherited, environmental factors also play a part in the development of allergic disorders. This is why not all members of a family, indeed not even both of a pair of identical twins, are affected to the same extent. Factors operating in early life, probably even during pregnancy, act together with the 'dose' of allergy genes that you inherited from your parents to determine whether or not allergy develops.

These early life factors include the timing of your first exposure to the allergen and the size of that exposure – however atopic you are, if you were never exposed to any allergen, you would not develop allergies. The number of viral infections suffered in early childhood may also have an effect – these infections seem to be protective against the development of allergy. High levels of exposure to tobacco smoke in pregnancy and early life increase an individual's risk of becoming atopic.

So, a baby born to cigarette smoking, cat-owning, atopic parents, whose birth coincides with the pollen season, who spends his or her first months in a well-insulated double-glazed house, and whose early life diet contains high levels of allergenic foods has a greatly increased risk of developing allergies.

WHY IS ALLERGY BECOMING MORE COMMON?

The single most important risk factor for developing allergic disease is being born to a mother or father who him- or herself has allergic disease. However, there has been a marked rise in the number of people suffering from allergies within just one generation and, as we know that changes in the genetic make-up of our population cannot occur that quickly, other factors must be involved. These include the following.

Infant feeding

If babies are exposed to food allergens such as cows' milk and eggs early in life they are more likely to develop allergic disease. Breast-feeding does not entirely protect the infant because allergens from food eaten by the mother can be secreted in breast milk.

Although current Department of Health guidelines suggest that solid food should not be introduced before the age of four months,

Environment

- Timing of first exposure to allergen

- Viral infection

- Tobacco smoke

- Allergenic foods

- Airborne allergens

- Household factors, e.g. dust mite

Genetic factors

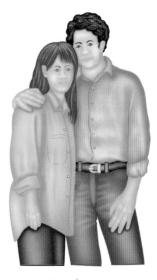

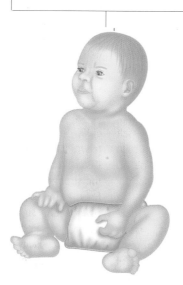

Allergies have a tendency to run in families. This is called atopy. Environmental factors also play a part in the development of allergic disorders. This is why not all members of a family are affected to the same extent.

many babies are started on solids rather earlier. The Western diet contains increasing amounts of commercially prepared food containing preservatives and other chemicals, and decreasing quantities of foodstuff such as fresh fruit and vegetables that contain protective antioxidants. Antioxidants are substances that slow down the breakdown of another substance by oxidation. They can also mop up free radicals, molecules that could otherwise damage healthy DNA. The most important antioxidants are vitamins A, C and E and selenium, with high levels being found in fresh fruit and vegetables.

Delaying the introduction of solid food appears to protect against allergies, especially eczema. The incidence of eczema by age two is directly related to the number of different solid foods taken by the baby before the age of four months. If a breast-feeding mother herself avoids highly allergenic food such as milk, eggs, peanuts and fish, an extra protective effect is seen.

Other allergens

Exposure to high levels of air-borne allergens in very early life appears to increase an infant's risk of developing allergic disease. Babies born in spring when the pollen count is high are more likely to be allergic to plant pollens at age ten than children born at other times of the year. Similarly, babies exposed to pet allergens in very early life have an increased risk of allergy. Although sensitisation may occur at any age, the first year of life appears to be particularly important, and there is increasing evidence to show that exposures in mid and late pregnancy are also important.

Tobacco smoke

Exposure to tobacco smoke both before (via the mother's bloodstream) and after birth is strongly associated with the development of allergies and allergic disease, particularly asthma. Babies born to smoking mothers have raised levels of IgE in their blood at birth. Exposure to smoke after birth increases the risk – children living in smoking households are twice as likely to be admitted to hospital with chest illness as children living in non-smoking households. These children also have significantly reduced lung function by age seven. Passive tobacco smoke exposure is the strongest identified risk factor for the development of allergic disease and so it is particularly alarming to see that smoking is still rising in popularity in young women of childbearing age.

Indoor environment

European children spend at least 90 per cent of their time indoors so the indoor environment is probably more important than all other geographical and outdoor environmental factors. Modern buildings tend to be well insulated and have poor levels of ventilation, and these factors appear to be a risk factor for the development of allergies. This may be the result of increased levels of chemical fumes from materials such as plastics and synthetic paints, high humidity leading to indoor mould growth and increased levels of house-dust mite allergen. These living conditions seem to exert a particularly powerful effect in atopic children – already at risk because of a family history of asthma.

Infections and antibiotics

Clear evidence is emerging that frequent viral and bacterial infections in early life may protect against the development of atopy and allergic diseases. Early life infections encourage the production of a chemical called interferon-gamma, which is found in higher levels in non-allergic people than in allergic people. If our children develop lower levels of interferon-gamma because we protect them from catching minor infections when they are young, we may be inadvertently increasing their chances of developing allergic disease. The overuse of antibiotics may have a similar effect.

In contrast, children who have large numbers of older brothers and sisters, and who go to child-care centres where they mix with large numbers of other children (and their germs), are less likely to develop hay fever and asthma.

IMMUNISATIONS

It is vital that we continue to protect our children from dangerous infections such as polio, tetanus, whooping cough, measles, mumps and rubella by the use of immunisations. Any benefit that might be given by not immunising is vastly outweighed by the harm done in leaving children vulnerable to catching these childhood infections; all of them are unpleasant and some can kill.

FINALLY

Our Western diet, with the use of formula milk and the early introduction of solid foods, in combination with our Western lifestyle (early life exposure to tobacco smoke, high levels of plant and animal allergens, house-dust mite, living in poorly ventilated humid houses, having smaller families and delayed use of child-care centres) all conspire to increase the number of children in our population developing allergic problems.

KEY POINTS

✓ An allergic reaction is an inappropriate and harmful response of your body's defence mechanisms to substances that are normally harmless

✓ Sensitisation does not always occur the first time that your body meets a particular allergen, and a substance may be tolerated for many years before an allergy develops

✓ Once you have become sensitised, even a tiny amount of allergen can produce an allergic response

✓ Although atopy (genetic tendency towards allergy) is inherited, environmental factors also play a part in the development of allergic disorders

Which medical problems are related to allergy?

A number of common conditions such as asthma, hay fever and eczema are allergic in nature. Also, there are less common but still important conditions, for example, urticaria and anaphylaxis, which are caused by allergens.

ASTHMA

Asthma is the most common chronic disease of childhood, affecting about one in seven children. Approximately one in ten adults also have asthma.

The normal airway has a delicate lining (epithelium) consisting of a number of different types of cells. These include cells that produce a lubricant (mucus) and cells with fine hair-like processes (cilia). The cilia move rhythmically to pass the mucus upwards towards the back of the throat, where it is swallowed. It carries with it with any dust particles that have been breathed in.

Beneath the epithelium is a layer called the submucosa. Beneath the submucosa is a sheet of muscle that wraps around the airway and which, when it contracts, makes the airways narrower.

Asthma is a chronic inflammation of the lining of the lung airways that leads to:

- swollen airway walls and narrowed air passages

- increased mucus production in the airways

- twitchy and oversensitive airway muscles.

Narrowed swollen airways make it more difficult for air to move in and out of the lungs. This leads to wheezing. The lining of the airways is irritable, leading to episodes of coughing. As the airway wall muscles are oversensitive, further

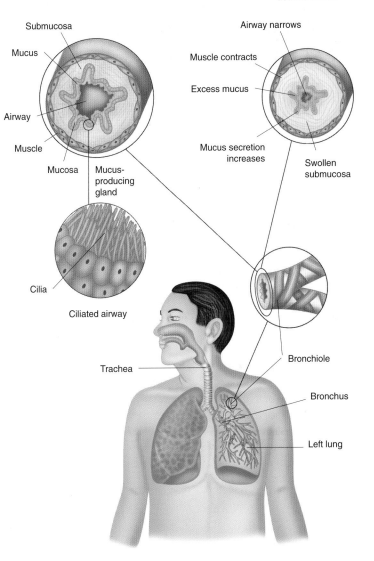

Normal airway

Submucosa

Mucus

Airway

Muscle

Mucosa

Mucus-producing gland

Cilia

Ciliated airway

Airway during asthma attack

Airway narrows

Muscle contracts

Excess mucus

Mucus secretion increases

Swollen submucosa

Trachea

Bronchiole

Bronchus

Left lung

During an asthma attack, the muscle walls of the airway contract, causing the internal diameter to narrow. Increased mucus secretions and inflammation of the airways' inner linings cause further narrowing.

airway narrowing can occur quite rapidly, producing sudden (acute) symptoms including breathlessness and chest tightness.

Sometimes symptoms are predictable, for example, when a person who is allergic to cats visits a cat-owning family. At other times, symptoms seem to occur for no particular reason.

Common triggers to symptoms include:

- allergens, for example, pet dander, house-dust mite, mould spores

- upper respiratory tract infections, for example, the common cold

- tobacco smoke

- high levels of air pollution

- sudden changes in air temperature

- exercise.

Many children with asthma are perfectly well and symptom free most of the time and develop asthma symptoms only when they meet one of their triggers. They then have an asthma attack, which may last a few hours or go on for days. Sometimes, long-term exposure to allergens or cigarette smoke can lead to persistent symptoms of asthma. Removing the trigger often leads to a marked improvement.

The pattern tends to be different in adults, who often have persistent (chronic) symptoms but also suffer sudden worsening of their asthma in the form of asthma attacks. Asthma can develop at any age, even in elderly people, in whom it is often confused with bronchitis, which is an infection of the airways.

HAY FEVER

Hay fever is a misleading term because hay has very little to do with causing the problem, and sufferers rarely have a fever. The medical term is seasonal allergic rhinitis – seasonal because it occurs only in certain months of the year and rhinitis meaning inflammation of the nose.

If you have hay fever, you are allergic to an allergen that is light enough to be carried in the air (an aeroallergen). A wide range of allergens can cause hay fever, including grass pollen, flower pollens and a wide variety of tree pollens. You can be allergic to more than one allergen, so your symptoms might vary throughout the hay fever season.

If your hay fever symptoms go on all year, then your condition is called perennial allergic rhinitis, and the likely culprit is the house-dust mite or perhaps a pet allergen, for example, cat or dog dander. Although it is not a life-threatening condition, hay fever causes a great deal of misery. It is also very common, affecting up to a quarter of the population at some time during the year.

The symptoms of hay fever come from a localised allergic reaction in the nose, throat and eyes. Once an allergy to a particular aeroallergen has been established, further contact with the allergen stimulates the cells of your immune system to release histamine and other chemicals, causing the small blood vessels in your nose, throat and eyes to enlarge and become leaky. Your eyes become itchy and watery, your nose becomes stuffed up and runny, and sneezing is a common problem. Some people find that they also have itchiness of the ears, which happens because a nerve links the back of the throat and the ears.

As your nose is often blocked, your senses of smell and taste are often affected. Swelling of the lining of your sinuses, the air-filled spaces in the bones of your face, can affect their drainage and cause sinusitis. On top of all these symptoms, sufferers often feel miserable, irritable and listless, and many people find their ability to work, drive and enjoy their social life is seriously impaired. Children with hay fever often find it

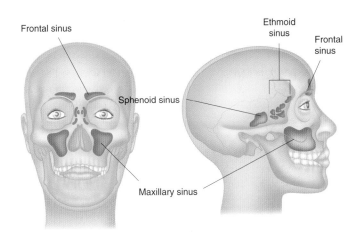

The sinuses are several air-filled cavities located in the skull bones around the eyes, cheeks and nose. Swelling of the lining of the sinuses can cause unpleasant symptoms.

COMMON SYMPTOMS OF HAY FEVER

- Sneezing
- A runny or stuffy nose
- Itching of the eyes, nose and throat
- Itching, watery and inflamed eyes (conjunctivitis)
- A dark appearance under the eyes due to inflammation in the sinuses
- Loss of sense of smell
- Tiredness, lethargy and irritability
- Asthma may become worse

difficult to perform well in end-of-year examinations which generally fall during the hay fever season.

Hay fever is rare in very young children. The most common time for it to start is between the ages of 6 and 25, and it is much less common in elderly people. Individuals who have previously suffered eczema or asthma are more at risk of developing hay fever.

THE SKIN: ECZEMA, DERMATITIS, URTICARIA AND ANGIO-OEDEMA

The skin is the largest organ of the body and every day is in direct contact with a vast array of different substances, including many allergens. It is not therefore surprising that the skin is frequently affected by allergic disease. There are four main skin problems caused by allergy: eczema, contact dermatitis, urticaria and angio-oedema.

Eczema

The correct name for eczema is atopic dermatitis. This is a chronic (long-lasting and recurring) inflammatory skin condition that occurs in atopic individuals (see page 17). Up to 15 per cent of children develop eczema in childhood; over 50 per cent of these children go on to develop asthma and 75 per cent of them develop hay fever.

Eczema usually occurs in children who have inherited a tendency for hypersensitivity or allergic reaction from their parents (atopy). A number of everyday factors can increase the likelihood of eczema developing. Exposure early in life to certain allergens such as eggs, cows' milk, pet dander and house-dust mite may increase the risk. At least 80 per cent of eczema sufferers have positive allergy tests to one or more allergens.

Eczema usually starts before the age of five years and, although it tends to improve over time, about 25 per cent of affected children continue to have eczema into adulthood.

Eczema causes itchy, red, raised lesions on the skin that can look blistered. They are often open and weeping as a result of scratching. Eventually the skin becomes thickened and scaly. The site of the lesions varies with age. The face, the outer surfaces of the arms and the knees are most affected in infants and young children; the neck, ankles and inner aspects of the knees and elbows are affected more in older children and adults. Persistent scratching can cause patchy changes in the pigmentation of the skin, which can look darker or lighter. Also, chronic infection of the

Typical example of atopic eczema

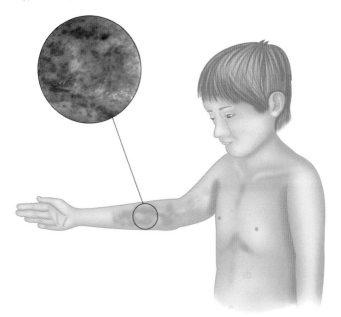

Eczema causes itchy, red, raised lesions of the skin that can look blistered. They are often open and weeping as a result of scratching.

Infants – whole body except bottom and groin

Children – neck, ankles, legs and arms

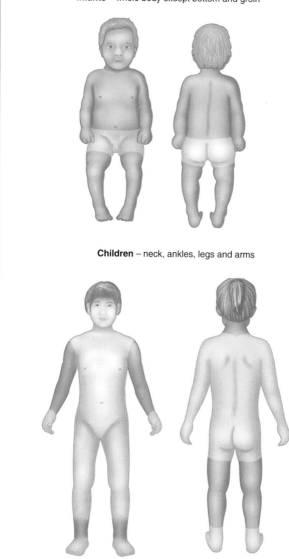

Adults – neck, ankles, inner aspects of the knees and elbows

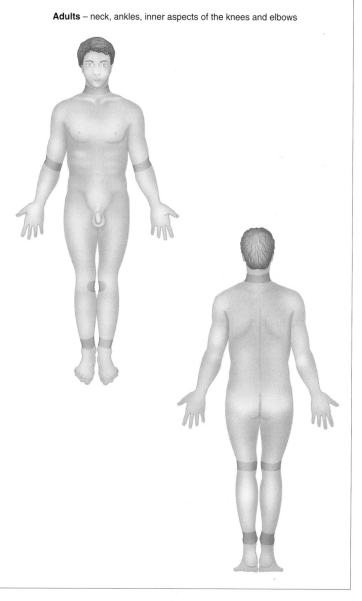

affected areas often occurs. The skin lesions follow a relapsing course, with bad episodes often being followed by periods when symptoms subside.

Once eczema has developed, certain triggers can make it worse. These include:

- diet – such as eating a trigger food

- chemicals – for example, in washing powders (particularly biological ones including enzymes), skin creams, soaps and shampoos

- stress and anxiety

- the weather – particularly cold weather

- airborne allergens such as pollen, pet allergens and house-dust mite.

Changing the type of your bedding, acquiring a new pet and the start of the pollen season can all make eczema worse. Also, manufacturers sometimes change the formulation of their products, so a product you have used without a problem in the past may suddenly cause your skin to get worse.

Allergic contact dermatitis

Contact dermatitis occurs when the skin is in contact with a chemical that can act as an irritant or an allergen. Most contact dermatitis is caused by irritants – any one of us can develop dermatitis if sufficient irritant is applied to our skin for long enough. Only about 20 per cent of all cases of contact dermatitis are caused by allergens and this problem is known as allergic contact dermatitis. This happens only in individuals who have been sensitised to that particular substance. Allergic contact dermatitis is more common in atopic individuals (see page 16), and is found most often in adults, being rare in children and elderly people. Sensitisation usually takes several days to develop. If the chemical is in contact with the skin again, a reaction will develop within 48 hours.

Allergic contact dermatitis is the most common work-related illness. People in certain jobs are more at risk, particularly hairdressers, cleaners and factory workers. It is more common in women, probably because they are repeatedly exposed to the chemicals found in household cleaners, and in people with fair skin.

The skin lesions in allergic contact dermatitis can look very similar to those in eczema. Blistering of the surface of the skin can be followed by thickening and scaling. There is often intense

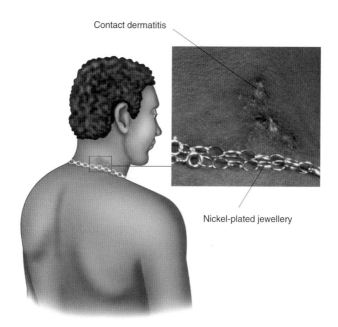

Contact dermatitis

Nickel-plated jewellery

Nickel allergy is probably the most common cause of allergic contact dermatitis.

itching. However, only the parts of the body exposed to the allergen are affected. Over half of all cases involve the hands. The outline of the area involved might suggest the cause – the round imprint of a watch on the wrist, a rectangle on the skin the same size as a sticking plaster, or a rash on the part of a face on which a particular cosmetic is used. This is in contrast to the lesions seen in eczema, which are not well demarcated.

Substances most commonly causing contact dermatitis are nickel, latex, soaps and detergents, food substances, preservatives, fragrances, lanolin, formaldehyde and potassium dichromate. Plants such as chrysanthemums and plant-derived materials such as latex may also be to blame. Nickel allergy is probably the most common cause of allergic contact dermatitis, with at least ten per cent of the population being affected. Nickel is found in jewellery, zips and jeans buttons.

Urticaria and angio-oedema
When an immediate allergic reaction happens in the skin, it becomes itchy and raised weals occur which look like nettle rash.

Redness and swelling around the weals can also be seen. These changes are caused by acute (rapid onset) allergic inflammation and are called urticaria. Acute urticaria affects as many as 20 per cent of the population at some time in their lives. It is usually short-lived and gets better without any treatment. In rare cases the urticaria can persist for weeks.

When the same type of reaction occurs in deeper layers of the skin, the reaction is called angio-oedema. In this there is little or no itching but the swelling might be quite painful. Although urticaria can happen virtually anywhere on the skin, angio-oedema usually involves the face and tongue.

A wide range of different factors can cause urticaria and angio-oedema. These include:

- direct contact with allergen, by skin contact, inhalation, injection or ingestion

- infections

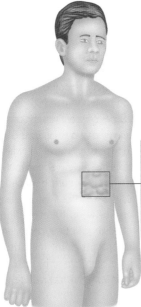

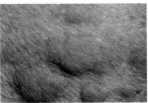

Example of urticaria

Urticaria.

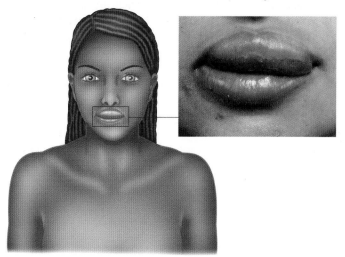

Example of angio-oedema

Angio-oedema.

- physical stimuli – such as cold, pressures, vibration and sunlight

- exercise (rarely).

FOOD ALLERGIES

Although unpleasant reactions to foods are common, not all of these are caused by allergy. As many as 20 per cent of the population believe that they are allergic to one or more foodstuffs, but on formal diagnostic testing, fewer than one in ten of these people have true food allergy. The rest are not imagining their symptoms, which are real – they may be caused by the food in question but it is not acting as an allergen.

Allergy, sensitivity and intolerance

In a large study enquiring about food allergy in 7,500 households, 20 per cent of households reported that at least one family member had food allergy. However, when these individuals were scientifically tested (using a double-blind, placebo-controlled challenge, see page 55) only between 1.4 and 1.8 per cent of adults had true food allergy. The symptoms in all the others may have been caused by food aversion, food intolerance or food sensitivity.

Food aversion

People with food aversion have had a previous unpleasant experience with a particular food and believe that whenever they eat the same food again they will have the same unpleasant reaction. This is not so, but because they believe it will happen they feel unwell even when they see or think of the food in question.

Food intolerance

In food intolerance, unpleasant symptoms occur after eating a food because your body cannot handle that food adequately. For example, some people have unpleasant symptoms of bloating, crampy abdominal pain and diarrhoea when they drink milk or eat products made from milk. This is because they do not produce sufficient quantities of the bowel enzyme that digests the milk sugar, lactose. Small quantities of milk can often be tolerated, but larger quantities lead to these symptoms. This is not because of allergy, in which even tiny amounts can lead to quite severe symptoms, but is the result of intolerance of lactose. Symptoms can be avoided by eliminating milk and milk products from the diet.

Food sensitivity

Food sensitivity occurs when you are more than usually sensitive to certain properties of a food. The type of reaction can be predicted from the food's chemical composition. For example, some people are very sensitive to the caffeine found in coffee and tea – they feel anxious and have marked tremor of their hands after taking small quantities.

It is important to distinguish intolerance, sensitivity, aversion and allergy, so that you receive the most effective form of treatment for your symptoms and understand how it may affect you in the future. For example, if you suffer from lactose intolerance your condition will probably stay with you all your life, whereas small children often outgrow their milk allergy.

What foods cause allergic reactions?

In young children, the most common food allergies are to cows' milk and eggs. In later childhood, fish, shellfish, peanuts and tree nuts are the most common allergens. Some allergies, particularly cows' milk allergy, may improve with time; others such as peanut allergy generally stay with you. Cows' milk allergy occurs in between two and five per cent of infants with up to 80 per cent of these infants losing their allergy by the age of five.

Children allergic to cows' milk are almost always allergic to sheep and goats' milk, and so these should not be used as a substitute. Soy-based milks should be used instead, and are well tolerated by most infants.

What are the symptoms?

Food allergy can cause a range of allergic symptoms in a number of different parts of the body:

- itchy nettle-like rash (urticaria)

- swelling of the lips, tongue and face (angio-oedema)

- wheezing and shortness of breath

- swelling of the larynx (voice box)

- breathing difficulties

- severe life-threatening collapse with shock (anaphylaxis).

All these symptoms occur within minutes of the exposure. Other symptoms can come on after a delay of a few hours, including:

- nausea

- abdominal pains

- vomiting and diarrhoea

- worsening of eczema.

Peanut allergy

The number of people affected by allergy to peanuts is rising. This problem has received a great deal of attention in the media in recent years, resulting at least in part from the small but increasing number of deaths caused by peanut allergy occurring in young people.

The peanut (*Arachis hypogea*) is not a true nut but a legume (a seed that grows in a pod, related to the lentil and pea families). Another name for it is ground nut. Peanuts are a cheap source of protein and are used widely in the world as food

FOOD ALLERGY

- Unpleasant reactions to foods are common and allergy is only one of many causes

- Symptoms of food allergy can range from mild itchy rashes to life-threatening anaphylaxis

- The most common foods causing allergy in the UK are cows' milk, hen's eggs, peanuts, fish and shellfish

- The best way of managing food allergy is to avoid the allergen

The nutritional panel on food packaging will help you avoid the substances causing your symptoms.

and as one of the largest sources of edible oil. Peanut oil is used in cooking, as well as in a wide range of cosmetic preparations such as soaps and shampoos, and in medical skin care products. In the past, peanut oil was used in many infant milk formulas but this practice has now been stopped.

The allergens responsible for peanut allergy are stable to heat and not inactivated by cooking. Although good quality distilled peanut (ground nut) oil does not contain any protein and is therefore not a risk for peanut-allergic patients, cold pressed oils can contain significant amounts of protein and can cause an allergic reaction. As peanuts are used in a wide range of foodstuffs, sensitisation can occur early in life. The resulting allergy is usually life long.

Allergic reactions to peanuts can be classed as mild, moderate or severe. If itchy skin rashes (hives, urticaria) are the only symptom, it is a mild reaction. A moderate reaction might involve swelling of the face, tightening of the throat and breathing difficulties other than wheezing. A severe reaction (called an anaphylactic reaction) would include wheezing, abdominal pain and collapse, with blueness of the lips and tongue. Peanut allergy is the most common cause of severe allergic reactions (anaphylaxis) in the USA and possibly also in the UK.

In 90 per cent of peanut-allergic individuals, the allergic reaction can be caused by a very small amount of peanuts (less than one nut). In over 50 per cent of sufferers, the symptoms start immediately after exposure and in 76 per cent within five minutes. In general, children suffer milder reactions than adults. Most peanut-allergic individuals suffer either mild or moderate reactions, severe reactions occurring in only seven per cent. Severe reactions are more common in those who also have asthma.

The best way of diagnosing peanut allergy is from the answers you give to questions about your medical past (your clinical history), in combination with skin-prick testing (see 'Diagnosing your allergies', page 50). The size of your reaction on skin-prick testing to peanuts is related to the severity of the reaction. Skin-prick testing is more sensitive than measuring the levels of specific antibodies (specific IgE) in your blood, and antibody levels do not tend to mirror the severity of the allergic reaction.

Once peanut allergy has been diagnosed, it is vital that all forms of peanuts are excluded from your diet. However, this is easier said than done! At least 50 per cent of people known to have peanut allergy have at least one accidental exposure each year. As a result of this, if you have peanut allergy you must AT ALL TIMES carry with you the right treatment to combat an allergic reaction (see 'Use of the EpiPen', page 47).

Sesame allergy

Sesame seeds are an extremely potent source of allergen. Sesame is used extensively in the food industry, both in its unprocessed form as a decoration for bread and other baked products and also in a wide range of processed foods, pharmaceutical products, toiletries and cosmetics. If you have sesame allergy, eating out may be a major problem – both the seeds and the oil produced from them must be avoided, and sesame oil is unrefined and may contain considerable amounts of sesame protein.

Sesame allergy was first reported in 1950 but initially very few cases were diagnosed. There has been a considerable rise in the numbers of people developing sesame allergy in the last decade. In one recent study of Australian children, sesame allergy was more common than allergy to tree nuts, although significantly less common than peanut allergy. Sesame allergy is believed to affect approximately one in every 2,000 people in the UK.

If you are allergic to sesame seeds, the mainstay of management is the avoidance of foods and other preparations containing sesame. Hummus, tahini and halvah are three popular sesame products. Sesame seeds in other food products can generally be identified from the labels. However, products containing 'vegetable oil' may contain sesame.

ALLERGIES AT WORK

Since the link was made between certain health problems and particular jobs, a number of Government Acts have tried to ensure that employees' working conditions are safe. A large number of health problems, some of which are allergic in origin, are still caused by contact with certain substances in the workplace. Allergies to such substances (occupational allergies) occur in both atopic and non-atopic individuals, being only slightly more common in those with asthma, eczema or hay fever. Many of the problem substances encountered at work do not cause allergy but act as irritants instead. These should be avoided by ensuring good workplace ventilation, by wearing or providing barrier clothing, or by substituting non-irritant alternatives.

There are over 200 substances that can cause allergic sensitisation leading to occupational asthma and at least as many causing skin allergies. Approximately 900,000 working days a year are lost in the UK because of occupational dermatitis. Occupational asthma accounts for two per cent of all adult asthma, with over 1,000 new cases per year.

Employers have a legal duty to protect their employees from hazards in the workplace and these include contact with allergic sensitisers. Providing that an occupational allergy is diagnosed early and from then on the problem substances avoided, there is a reasonable chance that the symptoms will disappear. However, if an allergy is allowed to become long standing, avoidance of the cause may improve the symptoms but they may not disappear completely. If you suspect that you have developed an occupational allergy, it is important for you to contact your work's doctor, your employment medical adviser or your general practitioner, so that you may be referred for further tests and specialist advice.

The most common substances causing allergy encountered in the workplace are latex, formaldehyde, soaps and detergents, food substances, potassium dichromate

HOW TO AVOID ALLERGIES IN THE WORKPLACE

- Avoid contact with materials that carry a manufacturer's hazard warning

- Avoid rough or abrasive work with your hands

- Always wash your hands properly after handling any potential irritant, but avoid getting your hands excessively wet, because damp skin is a less effective barrier

- Protect your hands from solvents, glue, grease, oil and corrosive chemicals by using barrier creams, after-wash creams and gloves

- Do not use solvents to remove substances from your hands as they themselves can cause dermatitis

- Use all protective apparatus supplied by your employer

- Avoid breathing in dust and fumes

- Report any problems to your line manager

- Encourage your colleagues to report their own work-related problems to their line manager

(found in many substances used in the building industry and in tanning leather), dye stuffs and the chemicals used in hairdressing.

DRUG ALLERGIES

There are a number of different ways in which drugs can cause adverse reactions. It is important to diagnose accurately whether or not allergy is responsible because the medical management and long-term outlook differ considerably.

Not all drugs can cause allergy. Those most frequently problematic are penicillin, other antibiotics, barbiturates, local anaesthetics and treatments that involve the injection of large molecules (such as insulin, some vaccines and some antisera made to treat the victims of bites by venomous creatures).

A drug allergy can take many forms, including urticaria, contact dermatitis (from topically applied drugs), anaphylaxis and severe generalised inflammation of the skin and the lining of the mouth and eyes (Stevens–Johnson syndrome).

A number of factors increase your risk of developing a drug allergy. These include:

- a current infection

- a family history of drug allergy

- a personal history of previous drug allergy

- diseases affecting your immune system, especially HIV

- a number of different drugs given in combination

- multiple courses or continuous use of a drug.

Although being atopic does not increase your likelihood of developing a drug allergy, it does increase your risk of having a severe reaction.

✓ Asthma is the most common chronic disease of childhood, affecting about one in seven children

✓ A wide range of allergens may be responsible for causing hay fever

✓ At least 80 per cent of eczema sufferers have positive allergy tests to one or more allergens

✓ Contact dermatitis occurs when the skin is exposed to an irritant or an allergen

✓ Urticaria and angio-oedema are two forms of immediate allergic reactions that happen in the skin

✓ As many as 20 per cent of the population believe that they are allergic to one or more foodstuffs, but only 10 per cent (one in ten) of these have true food allergy

✓ Once peanut allergy has been diagnosed, it is vital that all forms of peanuts are excluded from the diet

✓ Employers have a legal duty to protect their employees from hazards in the workplace and these include contact with allergic sensitisers

Anaphylaxis

naphylaxis is the most severe type of allergic reaction. It may involve a number of different systems of the body including the skin, the respiratory tract (mouth, nose, windpipe and lungs), the gastrointestinal tract (mouth, throat, stomach and intestine) and the cardiovascular system (heart and blood vessels). Anaphylactic reactions are potentially fatal, causing approximately 30 deaths per year in the UK, mainly in young adults.

SYMPTOMS

Anaphylactic reactions result from an exposure to an allergen to which a person is already sensitised. Instead of a localised reaction such as those described in the previous chapter, this further exposure produces a whole-body reaction. The widespread triggering of basophils and mast cells by IgE (see page 8) results in large-scale release of inflammatory mediators such as histamine and leukotrienes, which cause increased leakiness of the small blood vessels throughout the whole body. Fluid rapidly leaks from these small blood vessels into the tissues. This causes swelling within many body parts, which can interfere with normal body functioning, and loss of blood volume, causing blood pressure to fall. These changes result in the following symptoms:

- generalised itchiness, including itchiness of the skin, nose, eyes and throat

- flushing (reddening) of the skin

- urticaria and angio-oedema (see pages 31–3)

- hoarseness and difficulty in swallowing, because of swelling in the throat

- chest tightness and wheeze, caused by swelling and narrowing of the airways

- a fall in blood pressure causing a rapid weak pulse and a feeling of faintness

- nausea, vomiting and abdominal pain

- in severe cases, collapse and death.

TRIGGERS

The most common triggers to anaphylactic reactions are:

- bee and wasp stings

- foods, especially shellfish, peanuts, nuts, eggs and fish

- drugs, particularly antibiotics

- vaccines, especially tetanus anti-toxin.

Occasionally, physical stimuli such as exercise, heat, cold or anxiety may, usually in association with exposure to an allergen, cause anaphylaxis.

In a few cases, no cause of the anaphylactic reaction is discovered.

DIAGNOSIS

Once an individual has suffered a severe allergic reaction it is important to identify the trigger, because one of the main management strategies is the avoidance of that trigger in the future. In many cases a particular trigger will be strongly suspected and in others the cause will be a mystery, although careful questioning by an allergy expert will often unravel the cause. Skin-prick testing is the diagnostic test of choice – in most cases a direct challenge test is too dangerous in case it triggers a severe allergic reaction (see 'Diagnosing your allergies', page 50).

MANAGEMENT

Specialist clinics

Everyone who suffers anaphylaxis or a severe allergic reaction should be referred by the hospital in which they are treated or by their GP to an allergy specialist, who is a hospital consultant trained in the diagnosis and management of allergy. A list of allergy specialists is available from the British Society for Allergy and Clinical Immunology (see 'Useful addresses', page 95). People at particular risk of anaphylactic reactions are those who have asthma or other allergies. People with poorly controlled asthma are particularly at risk.

Trigger avoidance

If the trigger to anaphylaxis is known, it should be scrupulously avoided. If the trigger is a food, the help of a dietitian may be very useful in helping you to avoid that food in the future. Your GP or allergy specialist can refer you to a dietitian. Even very small traces of the problem food can trigger a reaction, and in severe cases skin contact with the allergen or breathing in air containing tiny particles of it may be enough to cause a reaction.

• **Peanuts:** This is discussed more in the section 'Peanut allergy' (see page 35).

• **Eggs:** Egg is found in a wide variety of processed foods. It is important to read the contents list carefully – it may be described by a number of names, including albumin, egg white and dried egg. Eggs are often used as glazing on baked goods.

WHAT YOU SHOULD DO IF YOU ARE STUNG BY A BEE OR WASP – MILD-TO-MODERATE REACTIONS

Keep calm, and if possible do not walk or run around because this will rapidly spread the poison around the body and put you at more risk of a severe reaction.

If the sting remains embedded in your skin, remove it with tweezers, making sure not to squeeze the poison sac, which is a dark pouch that is at the back of the sting.

Cool the affected area, if possible with an ice pack or packet of frozen vegetables (cover the ice pack with a towel or tea towel, otherwise it might burn your skin).

For pain, take a pain-killer such as paracetamol or ibuprofen (ibuprofen is an anti-inflammatory as well as a pain-killer so is preferable, but take whichever you have to hand). If you develop anything more than mild local swelling, take an antihistamine (available over the counter from your chemist).

If the reaction doesn't subside and you develop more severe symptoms, follow your emergency treatment plan (see page 46).

- **Milks:** Milk is found in many foods as well as in the form of a drink. Words used to describe milk include whey, casein, caseinates, lactose, dry milk solids and milk powder. You must avoid butter, cheese, cream, yoghurt, crème fraiche, fromage frais, condensed milk, evaporated milk, ice cream, margarines and low-fat spreads, and milk chocolate – and any food that lists any of these as ingredients.

- **Insect stings:** There are many practical things that you can do to reduce the risk of being stung (see 'Treatment of allergic disease', page 62).

TREATMENT FOR ALLERGIC REACTIONS

Antihistamine medications

These should be taken as soon as you realise you are having an allergic reaction. Common preparations include chlorpheniramine (Piriton), cetirizine (Zirtek) and loratadine (Clarityn). These drugs block the effect of histamine, a substance released by the mast cells, which causes many of the symptoms of allergy – they may prevent a full-blown anaphylactic reaction from developing.

Epinephrine (adrenaline)

In the UK, the name adrenaline has been superseded by epinephrine. If you are at risk of an anaphylactic reaction you should carry epinephrine for injection with you at all times. Epinephrine works quickly when injected to counteract the effects of the chemicals released during an anaphylactic reaction by narrowing the small blood vessels, increasing the blood volume, stimulating the heart and increasing the blood pressure. You should always carry two devices because the effects of the first injection may begin to wear off before you reach medical help and you might need a second injection. In most situations two doses will be sufficient to buy you enough time to seek urgent medical help, but a third dose, if available, would do no harm.

You should know how to administer the injections, and should also teach relatives and close friends. In the case of a child, all the child's carers (including school-teachers) should know how and when to administer the epinephrine. Epinephrine and antihistamines can be used together without problems.

The most commonly used device for injectable epinephrine in the UK is the EpiPen. This is very easy to use, and you should carry your two pens with you everywhere you go. The best way to do this is to 'wear' them in some way – in a pocket or a bumbag – rather than putting them in a bag, which you might leave behind at times during the day.

EMERGENCY TREATMENT PLAN

You should prepare an emergency treatment plan so that you and those around you know exactly what to do if you experience a severe allergic reaction. Don't think this won't happen to you. Approximately half of those at risk of anaphylaxis are accidentally exposed to the trigger allergen that could cause a life-threatening allergic reaction each year. If you act quickly, you will be able to reduce the severity of the reaction greatly.

Carry with you an **information card** with your name, a brief description of your allergy and what treatment you may need if you have a severe allergic reaction, your address and emergency contact numbers for close relatives. Make it clear that you have a SERIOUS medical problem and state that anyone helping you should call an ambulance by dialling 999 immediately. You may also wish to wear a piece of medical identification jewellery (see 'Treatment of allergic disease', page 62 and 'Useful addresses', page 94).

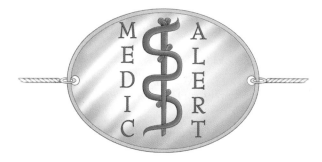

Example of medical identity jewellery

You should carry a copy of this plan with your emergency drug. Further copies should be given to appropriate colleagues and carers such as work colleagues, teachers and close friends. Special plans should be devised for children with severe allergy, and sample plans are available from the Anaphylaxis Campaign and Allergy UK (see 'Useful addresses', page 94).

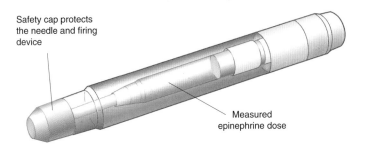

Safety cap protects the needle and firing device

Measured epinephrine dose

The most commonly used device for injectable epinephrine in the UK is the EpiPen.

If you think you may be developing a severe allergic reaction, use your epinephrine pen EARLY. Do not wait until you are sure – the dose of epinephrine will do you no harm, even if you turn out to be wrong and you do not develop a reaction. However, failing to use epinephrine when you should puts you at risk of having the worst kind of allergic reaction, which could kill you. If in doubt, use the epinephrine!

USE OF THE EPIPEN

- Pull off the grey safety cap

- Place the black tip on your upper outer thigh (it is not necessary to remove your clothes unless they are very thick and bulky)

- Press the EpiPen firmly against your thigh until you hear or feel the injector firing

- Hold the pen in place for 10 seconds

- Remove the pen and massage the injection site gently

- After using the EpiPen, seek medical advice *immediately*

- If allergic symptoms do not start to improve, give a second injection of epinephrine

- Carry your EpiPen with you at all times

Tips and precautions

Keep your EpiPen auto-injector at room temperature until the marked expiration date, at which point your unit should be replaced. It should not be refrigerated; refrigeration for extended periods may cause the unit to malfunction. Nor should the EpiPen auto-injector be exposed to extreme heat, such as in the glove compartment or trunk of a car during the summer.

Do not expose your auto-injector to direct sunlight; light and heat can cause epinephrine to degrade, turning brown. This shortens the usable life of the product.

The best way to protect your auto-injector is to keep it in the plastic tube it comes in.

Check your EpiPen auto-injector periodically through the viewing window of the unit to make sure the solution is clear and colourless. If the solution appears brown, replace the unit immediately.

Regardless of the colour of the epinephrine, always replace your auto-injector with a fresh unit before the expiry date.

Seek medical help

If you need to use adrenaline you should call an ambulance IMMEDIATELY. A mobile phone may be a useful extra to have with you. Even though your prompt recognition and treatment of the allergic reaction may prevent anaphylaxis developing, you must go to an accident and emergency department where you will be observed for at least four hours to make sure that the reaction does not progress. Remember, the effects of epinephrine do not last long – after 30 minutes you may need another dose. As each EpiPen contains only one dose of epinephrine, once you have used a pen you must get a new one from your doctor immediately.

KEY POINTS

✓ Anaphylaxis is the most severe type of allergic reaction

✓ The most common triggers to anaphylactic reactions are foods (especially shellfish, peanuts, nuts, eggs and fish), bee and wasp stings, and drugs (particularly antibiotics)

✓ Everyone who suffers anaphylaxis or a severe allergic reaction should be referred to an allergy specialist

✓ If the trigger to anaphylaxis is known, it should be scrupulously avoided

✓ Prepare and carry an emergency treatment plan

✓ Carry your EpiPen with you at all times

Diagnosing your allergies

If you think you might have an allergy, it is important that your problem is accurately diagnosed. If it is an allergy, the correct treatment can be prescribed and a management plan worked out. If the problem is not the result of an allergy, you are then free to find out what the real cause is. This chapter describes each of the different allergy tests, with details of when each test might be needed and a discussion of their advantages and disadvantages.

Your doctor will almost certainly want to do at least one test. If you have suffered an allergic reaction but do not know what the cause was, the test will attempt to discover the allergen responsible. Even if you know the cause of your allergic reaction, the diagnosis may need to be confirmed by some form of allergy test, particularly if the allergic reaction was severe. The treatment for an allergic condition may involve long-lasting, time-consuming or expensive treatments and so it is as well to verify the cause beforehand. Allergy tests can also be helpful if there is any confusion about whether your problem is caused by a true allergy or whether it might be caused by an intolerance or sensitivity. Workplace allergies may have legal implications, and must always be verified by formal allergy testing.

The results of allergy tests must be interpreted by an expert, who will also consider the precise details of your problem. This is because allergy tests do not always provide a clear yes/no answer – rather they provide a clue in the clinical puzzle. As a result of this, I would not recommend that you have allergy tests performed by a commercial organisation because they are unable to interpret the results in the light of your clinical history and advise you appropriately.

Choosing the right test

Which test is right for you will depend on the details of your allergic reaction – for example, how old you are, which part of your body is affected, what the likely cause is, how severe the reaction is.

Every test used for diagnosing your allergies must be:

- relevant (includes the likely culprits)

- standardised (so that the results done in one centre can be related to those done in another)

- repeatable (so that results done on different occasions will be similar)

- specific (the test is positive only in people with that allergy)

- sensitive (the test does not falsely show as negative a test that should be positive).

No single allergy test is perfect, but by choosing the correct tests for each individual, the majority of allergic problems can be accurately diagnosed. If your problem proves particularly difficult to sort out, you should ask your doctor to refer you to an allergy specialist. This is the only way you can be referred to a specialist. A list of allergy specialists in the UK can be obtained from the British Society for Allergy and Clinical Immunology (see 'Useful addresses', page 95).

Skin-prick tests

Direct skin testing is the most commonly used diagnostic test for allergy. The skin test is a way of challenging you with an allergen using a safe and localised test and is a very sensitive way to demonstrate the presence of a true allergic reaction. Skin-prick testing is very safe and adverse events are extremely rare. However, individuals at high risk of experiencing a severe allergic reaction should be skin tested in a hospital setting. You must tell the person doing the skin tests if you are on any medications because treatment with antihistamines, corticosteroids and certain antidepressants may interfere with the tests. Skin testing can also be unreliable in very young and elderly people.

Skin tests are usually done on the inside aspect of your forearm, but the skin of the back is often used in small children. The sites for testing are marked with a pen and a single drop of a concentrated extract of the chosen allergen is placed at each site. The surface layer of your skin is gently punctured through the drop using a sterile lancet (an instrument with a small sharp prong 1 millimetre long). Any allergen left on your skin

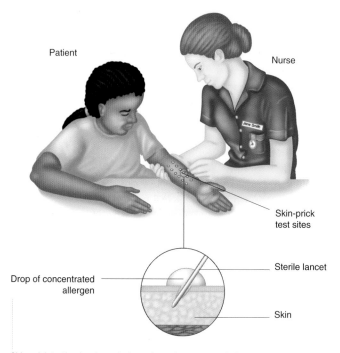

Patient

Nurse

Skin-prick
test sites

Sterile lancet

Drop of concentrated
allergen

Skin

Skin-prick testing involves placing a drop of concentrated allergen on the skin. The skin
is then punctured through the drop. A positive reaction to the allergen is shown by a
pale raised bump.

is then blotted with an absorbent tissue and after 10 minutes the diameters of the resulting reactions are measured. The whole process is repeated for each allergen being tested.

A positive result is shown by a weal (a pale raised bump), which may be itchy and may be surrounded by an area of red skin. As well as testing with allergens, two further pricks are done using a saline solution (negative control) and a histamine solution (a positive control) in order to test the reliability of the procedure. The response to the saline solution should be negative in everyone. If you have a positive result this shows that your skin is very sensitive and that testing will not be reliable. The response to histamine should be positive in everyone. If you have a negative result, your skin is being prevented from reacting normally, perhaps because of a drug you are taking and, again, testing will not be reliable.

Skin-prick testing is painless, and even young children tolerate the procedure very well. Positive reactions may be itchy but generally last less than an hour.

Skin-prick testing is a very sensitive test, so if you have a negative reaction you can be fairly certain you do not have that allergy. However, a positive reaction does not always mean that you have a current allergy. It may be that you have a hidden or latent allergy which is not causing you problems now but which might have done so in the past or may do so in the future.

Skin-prick testing is a simple, quick and inexpensive form of testing and many different allergens

can be tested at the same time, although there might not be enough space on your arm for more than 16.

Patch testing

This test is used in cases of contact dermatitis where allergy is suspected. It is generally performed on the skin of your back, and it is important that an area of clear skin, free of any disease, is used. It is a relatively simple and safe form of testing but, in severe cases, itching or blistering may develop as a response to the tests. Test allergens in appropriate concentrations are mixed with white soft paraffin

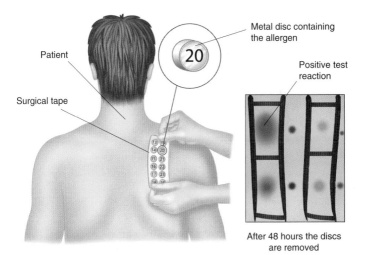

A patch test puts test allergens into small metal discs that are taped on to the skin of the back. The discs are left for 48 hours and then removed, and the underlying skin examined for reaction.

(which allows them to penetrate the skin surface more easily) and then spread on to metal discs the size of a one pence piece. These discs are placed on your skin, covered with an adhesive dressing and left in place for 48 hours. The discs are then removed and discarded and your skin is examined for any redness, swelling or blistering. Your skin is then re-examined after a further 48 hours.

The interpretation of the results of this form of testing is not easy, and requires a thorough knowledge of the materials being used and of your personal allergy history. When carefully done, patch testing can provide very helpful information for the diagnosis of contact dermatitis.

Specific IgE measurements

Specific allergy antibodies (IgE) can be measured in the blood using a radioallergosorbent test (RAST). This test can confirm that your immune system has produced increased levels of IgE against a suspected allergen, for example, house-dust mite. For this test, a small blood sample must be taken from a vein, usually from your arm, using a fine needle and small syringe. The sample is analysed by a specialist

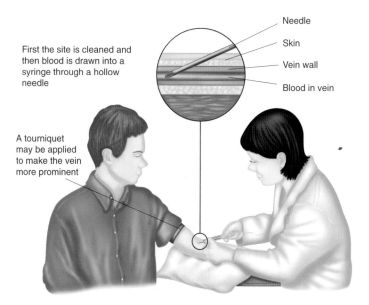

First the site is cleaned and then blood is drawn into a syringe through a hollow needle

Needle

Skin

Vein wall

Blood in vein

A tourniquet may be applied to make the vein more prominent

Specific allergy antibodies can be measured in the blood using a RAST to confirm that your immune system has produced increased levels of IgE against a suspect allergen.

laboratory, which can generally provide results within a few days.

This test is particularly useful when skin-prick testing is impossible, perhaps because the patient is unable to stop their antihistamine medications without their allergic disease getting very much worse. Extensive eczema or dermatitis also makes skin-prick testing impractical. Again, careful interpretation of the results of RAST is important because positive tests can occur in people without an allergy, and negative tests can occasionally occur in people who do have that specific allergy.

Challenge tests

Occasionally the best way of diagnosing and confirming an allergy is to provoke an allergic reaction by deliberately exposing the person to the suspected allergen, but by doing this in a careful and controlled way. The allergen should be given in an appropriate way, for example, if wheezing or asthma is the problem, the allergen should be inhaled. If food allergy is suspected, the test should be given by mouth. These forms of testing should never be used in a patient who has suffered a severe allergic reaction or anaphylaxis to the allergen.

Ideally both allergen and dummy (placebo) substances should be used and neither the individual being tested nor the tester should know which is which – this is called a 'double-blind placebo-controlled' challenge. A third person prepares the substances and keeps the records. The test is done in this way so that no-one involved in the tests can be influenced by any prior beliefs that they might have.

This form of test can be used when food allergy is suspected but the cause is not clear. For example, when several different foods have given a positive result on skin-prick testing, it might be unclear which of these foods is causing your symptoms. The results of a double-blind food challenge are usually very clear and, if a food does not give rise to symptoms, allergy can generally be ruled out. This type of test should NEVER be attempted at home, because it may result in a severe allergic reaction.

Lung function testing

Various forms of lung function tests can be used in making the diagnosis of asthma and in monitoring a patient's progress, particularly after changes in treatment.

The most common form of testing is the measurement of peak expiratory flow. Peak expiratory flowmeters (peak flowmeters) are small hand-held devices that measure the flow of air from your lungs. The harder you are able to blow, the higher the reading. If you have asthma, your peak flow levels are likely to be lower than those of someone with normal lungs, but, in addition, they will vary more from one day to another. As a result of this, you will usually be asked to record your peak flows, both morning and evening, for at least one week, and often longer.

If you are used to recording your peak flows, the measurements can be particularly useful in helping you judge whether your asthma is going out of control and whether you need to increase your medication. Peak flow can also be helpful in people who find it difficult to judge how bad their asthma is.

Peak flowmeters provide information that can be extremely helpful in the day-to-day management of asthma. You and your doctor can agree on a plan that allows you to judge the amount of treatment you require based on your symptoms and your peak flow readings. You can then manage change in your symptoms without having to ask for medical help every time.

SYMPTOM DIARIES

Occasionally your doctor might ask you to keep a record of your symptoms on a daily basis along with details of the factors suspected of causing them. This will help you and your doctor to see the relationship between various triggers and your symptoms. As allergy often causes intermittent problems, you may be completely well on the days on which you see your doctor. A symptom diary is an accurate way of telling your doctor how frequent and how serious your symptoms are, and may give clues as to what the causes might be.

It can be quite hard work to keep a detailed symptom diary, because it may take many weeks to record sufficient details to provide the necessary information. Symptom diaries will always be subjective, but you must be as honest as possible and put down everything that you think important. Used in conjunction with a full symptom history, symptom diaries can often provide very useful clues in identifying the cause of allergic symptoms.

TRIAL OF TREATMENT

Sometimes allergic disease can be quite difficult to diagnose accurately, and a useful way of clinching a diagnosis is to commence appropriate anti-allergy treatment and to see whether or not your symptoms improve. This is known as a trial of treatment. Of course your doctor would weigh up the potential risks against the potential benefits and would not start any treatment unless it was safe to do so. In this situation a symptom diary (or a peak

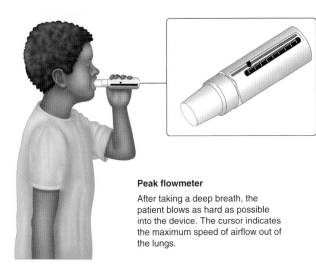

Peak flowmeter

After taking a deep breath, the patient blows as hard as possible into the device. The cursor indicates the maximum speed of airflow out of the lungs.

You will usually be asked to record your peak flows both morning and evening for at least a week, on charts similar to those shown below.

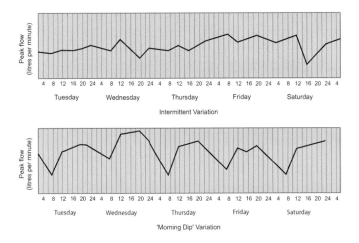

The most common form of lung function test is the measurement of peak expiratory flow using a peak flowmeter that measures the flow of air from your lungs. The harder you blow, the higher the reading.

Date this card was started:	1	2	3	

1. ASTHMA LAST NIGHT

Slept well all night...0

Awoke early, or once in night with cough or wheeze....1

Awoke 2–4 times...2

Awake for most of the night with cough or wheeze......3

2. WHEEZE AND BREATHLESSNESS TODAY

None...0

Mild, but not troublesome...1

Troublesome..2

Severe...3

3. DURING EXERCISE – HOW MUCH ACTIVITY COULD YOU MANAGE TODAY?

Able to walk, run and play without cough
or breathlessness...0

Normal when walking. Cough or breathlessness
when running..1

Slight cough or breathlessness even when walking. 2

Severe cough or breathlessness when
walking. Unable to run..3

4. PEAK FLOWMETER (best of three blows standing up) Before breakfast medicine

Before bedtime medicine

5. DRUGS	Name of drug	Dose	1	2	3	
Number of occasions taken in past 24 hours						

	6	7	8	9	10	11	12	13	14	15	16	17	18	19	20	21

	6	7	8	9	10	11	12	13	14	15	16	17	18	19	20	21

flowmeter in the case of asthma) can be extremely useful in monitoring the effect of the treatment.

Sometimes, instead of the treatment taking the form of a drug or medication, a change in your environment or the avoidance of a particular allergen might be indicated. There are more details about allergen avoidance in the next chapter.

TESTS USED BY ALTERNATIVE ALLERGY SPECIALISTS

Specialists in alternative or complementary medicine sometimes use tests that are not used in a conventional medical assessment. These have not been scientifically evaluated using well-conducted clinical studies. Many of them are not based on any accepted scientific theory. Complementary therapists claim these tests give useful information, but these claims are not backed up by any evidence and orthodox doctors are not convinced of their value. Examples are: applied kinesiology, cytotoxic testing, provocation–neutralisation, Vega testing, hair analysis and pulse tests.

Applied kinesiology

Muscle strength is measured both before and after exposure to a suspected allergen trigger. This test is based on the theory that allergy impairs the strength of skeletal muscle.

Cytotoxic test

This test is based on an as yet unproven theory that a food allergy alters the shape and size of white blood cells.

Provocation–neutralisation technique

In this test, increasing doses of a substance suspected of causing an allergy are administered under your tongue or as subcutaneous injections until you experience a 'sensation', thought to represent an allergic response. The nature or intensity of the symptoms or sensations are not standardised and need not be the same as the symptoms being investigated. Further concentrations of the substance are then given until you report the disappearance of symptoms.

Vega testing

This measures the electromagnetic fields that you produce both before and after you are in physical contact with an allergen.

Hair analysis

Your hair is examined and its appearance and chemical content is used to diagnose a range of medical problems.

Pulse test

A change in your pulse rate after exposure to an allergen has been claimed by some to be diagnostic of allergy to that substance. This test is usually used in cases of suspected food allergy.

None of these tests has been shown to be of any medical value.

KEY POINTS

✓ Accurate diagnosis of allergic problems is very important

✓ The results of allergy tests must be interpreted by an expert

✓ Skin testing is a simple, quick and inexpensive form of testing

✓ Patch testing is used in cases of contact dermatitis where allergy is suspected

✓ RAST is particularly useful when skin-prick testing is impossible

✓ Peak flowmeters provide information that can be extremely helpful in the day-to-day management of asthma

✓ A symptom diary is an accurate way of telling your doctor how frequent and how serious your symptoms are

✓ Alternative or complementary medicine practitioners sometimes use tests that have not been scientifically evaluated

Treatment of allergic disease

GENERAL PRINCIPLES

Once allergy has been found to be the cause of your problem, the next step is to reduce your symptoms to a minimum by finding an appropriate treatment. Most people with allergic problems will need to use one or more medications to control their condition. However, if you can identify the responsible allergen, it may be possible to reduce your exposure to it or to avoid it completely, and by doing so you may be able to reduce markedly your need for drug treatment. Other more general measures may also help, such as maintaining good general health, eating a healthy diet, and avoiding exposure to tobacco smoke and other sources of air pollution. Finally, you may be a suitable candidate for immunotherapy (see page 77), a treatment that aims to damp down or even eliminate the allergy, although this is not appropriate for everyone.

The aims of treatment are to:

- reduce symptoms, particularly the frequency and severity of acute episodes

- minimise restrictions in lifestyle

- improve quality of life including the ability to enjoy work, leisure, exercise, eating, socialising and sleeping

- reduce time lost from school and work

- improve self-esteem.

Allergen avoidance

The best treatment for an allergy is to avoid completely whatever it is that triggers your symptoms, namely the allergen(s) to which you are allergic. This is relatively easy if your allergy is to something like nickel. However, there are some allergens that are impossible to avoid completely – for example, pollen and house-dust mite.

Don't despair! There are a number of practical ways in which you can reduce your contact with many allergens and in doing so reduce your need for drug treatment. We are not yet able to cure allergies but, by a combination of allergen avoidance and the right medical treatment, the symptoms of your allergy should be kept under good control.

Indoor airborne allergens

We now spend over 90 per cent of our lives indoors. Most of the air we breathe therefore comes from the indoor environment. Allergy to indoor allergens can be found in at least two of three patients with asthma, allergic rhinitis and eczema. The most common indoor allergens are:

- the house-dust mite

- cat dander

- dog dander

- moulds and spores

- cockroach (in some countries).

All of these allergens, combined with other factors, may make the symptoms of asthma, allergic rhinitis and eczema worse. Not only do we now spend more time inside our houses but modern houses themselves create an ideal environment for the collection of high levels of indoor allergens. Over the last 30 years houses have become warmer, with reduced levels of ventilation as a result of draught exclusion, double-glazing and the elimination of open fireplaces. As a consequence of the lack of ventilation and the higher temperatures, humidity within the home has increased. In addition, fitted carpets and soft furnishings act as reservoirs for allergens and the use of efficient detergents for clothes washing has led to the use of cooler wash temperatures that are less effective at destroying allergens that might be carried on clothing.

House-dust mite allergy

House-dust mite allergy is the most common allergy in both children and adults in the UK. House-dust mites are microscopic eight-legged insects that live on a diet of human skin scales. They grow and reproduce best in warm, humid conditions such as those found in carpets, mattresses, sofas and clothing. It is the mite's faecal (waste) particles that contain the allergen.

House dust contains large quantities of mites and their faecal particles. The house-dust mite is rare in cold countries, at high altitude and in the hospital environment. As a result of this, the symptoms of house-dust mite allergy are likely to improve at altitude and when in hospital.

Before you spend a lot of time, energy and money trying to reduce the levels of house-dust mite in your home, you should first find out whether or not you are allergic to them. This can be done by skin-prick testing or by a blood test (see pages 51 and 54). If you do have a house-dust mite allergy, it is worth trying to reduce your exposure to this allergen. You can do this in the following ways.

• **Vacuuming:** Vacuum clean regularly using a high efficiency vacuum cleaner fitted with an efficient filter with a pore size of less than 0.3 micrometres (all manufact-urers now give details of the filters they fit). Many of the ordinary vacuum cleaners currently available meet this specification, so it is not necessary to buy an expensive 'medical' vacuum cleaner.

The information you will need to make your choice is available both from the manufacturers and from Allergy UK, which assesses many products including vacuum cleaners. If products meet their specifications, they award it their 'seal of approval'. As well as carpets, vacuum your mattress, curtains and any soft furnishings such as sofas, upholstered chairs and padded headboards (see 'Upholstery and soft furnishings' on page 66).

• **Bedding:** There are two possible approaches here. One is to keep your bedding as allergen free as possible by regularly washing your pillows and duvet at a high temperature (at least 60°C in order to kill the house-dust mites and destroy their allergen) and by regularly vacuuming the mattress. The other approach is to place a barrier between you and your bedding. Using barrier covers is probably the easiest way to tackle your mattress, duvet and pillow. Even if these items are full of house-dust mites, putting an efficient barrier between you and them (and their waste droppings) will prevent your symptoms being triggered.

The cheapest solution is to use plastic covers, which should completely enclose the item. Remember to seal over the top of the zip fasteners with adhesive tape. However, these plastic covers are uncomfortable as they can feel rather hot and damp and are also noisy.

More expensive anti-allergy covers are available. They are made from microporous breathable material and their cost has come

BEDS AND BEDDING

Beds and bedding make an ideal environment for house-dust mites to live in. It is worth taking some protective measures to reduce your prolonged and regular exposure if you are sensitised to this allergen.

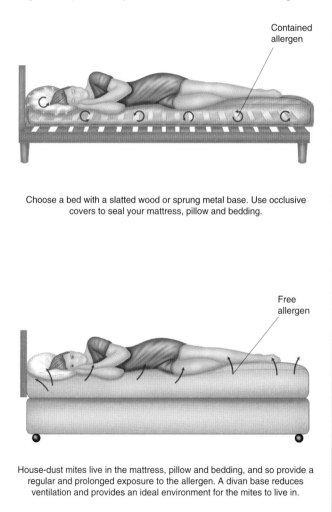

Contained allergen

Choose a bed with a slatted wood or sprung metal base. Use occlusive covers to seal your mattress, pillow and bedding.

Free allergen

House-dust mites live in the mattress, pillow and bedding, and so provide a regular and prolonged exposure to the allergen. A divan base reduces ventilation and provides an ideal environment for the mites to live in.

down a lot in recent years. Allergy UK can provide you with details of manufacturers of items that carry the Allergy UK seal of approval. It is important to buy the whole system, including a pillow, duvet and mattress cover, otherwise the benefit will be extremely limited. As these covers are still not cheap, it is important that you confirm your house-dust mite allergy by having the appropriate tests.

Choose a bed with a slatted wood or sprung metal base. Avoid sleeping in a bed with a divan base because this makes an ideal home for the house-dust mite, and avoid sleeping on a lower bunk bed or on a bed with a canopy because you will be under a continual shower of house-dust mite allergen.

• **Carpets:** We spend more time in the bedroom than in any other room, so it makes sense to concentrate your efforts here. Ideally, all carpets should be removed from your bedroom and replaced with lino or wood flooring. If you do choose to have a carpet, it is better to have a synthetic carpet because these produce a static charge that attracts the mite particles to it and so reduces the amount of allergen in the air. Vacuum the carpets and the rest of the house regularly with a high efficiency vacuum cleaner.

• **Upholstery and soft furnishings:** All upholstered items should be removed from your bedroom. Ideally your bedroom curtains should be unlined and made of a thin washable material. Roller blinds are a good alternative. Large pieces of upholstered furniture can be heat-treated by enclosing them in a plastic cover and heating the air inside to 100°C. This treatment kills live house-dust mites and also destroys the allergen in their faecal particles (see 'Useful addresses', page 94).

• **Cuddly toys:** The number of cuddly toys in the bedroom should be reduced to an absolute minimum. Any essential cuddlies should be washed regularly at a temperature of at least 60°C. Although putting these toys in the freezer will kill the living house-dust mites, it will do nothing to remove the large amount of house-dust mite allergen that can be inside, so a hot wash is preferable. If cuddly toys have to be stored in the bedroom, you should put them in a plastic box with a tightly fitting lid.

• **Humidity and ventilation:** Increasing the ventilation of your home will reduce the humidity and so reduce the numbers of house-dust mites. The easiest way to do this is to open the windows. A small number of air filtration systems and ionisers have been shown to lower allergen levels in the home. Allergy UK (see Useful addresses on page 95) can recommend effective products.

• **House-dust mite sprays:** There are a number of sprays available that kill house-dust mites. However, in practice these are rarely effective because the spray can penetrate only a few millimetres into furnishings. In addition, the fumes from these sprays can irritate the eyes, skin and lungs.

Pet allergens

Between 60 and 80 per cent of households in the UK have a pet of some kind – cats are the most popular. At least a third of people with allergies are allergic to pet allergens – so they are a major trigger factor in allergic disease.

It is not necessary to handle an animal to come into contact with its allergen. The allergen can travel in small particles in the air and can be passed from person to person or from house to house on clothing and footwear. The allergen can be found in the fur and skin scales, the saliva, urine and faeces of the animal. No matter where in the home the pet lives, the allergen will quickly become distributed around the rest of the house, and so it is not enough to restrict the pet to certain parts of the home. Animal allergens persist for a long time and, once a pet has left a home, it may take many months of hard work with an efficient vacuum cleaner to remove most of the allergen.

If you are allergic to pet allergen, the obvious answer is not to keep that pet. However, we are a nation of animal lovers and some families are very reluctant to let their pet go. If you decide you want to keep your pet, try to keep your contact with the animal to a minimum. Maybe it can live outside or in the garage and never come into the house. When you stroke or handle the animal you should wear special clothing which you do not bring into the house. Leave the clothing in the garage or put it straight into the washing machine. Use a high efficiency vacuum cleaner regularly to remove as much of the allergen as possible from the home.

Consider washing your cat regularly – although this is easier said than done! Studies have shown that washing a cat once a week, particularly if you ask your vet for a special shampoo, significantly reduces the amount of allergen they shed.

Pollen

Plants can be pollinated in two ways, either by insects or by wind. It is the wind-pollinated plants that cause trouble for the sufferer of seasonal allergic rhinitis (hay fever).

GENERALISED POLLEN CALENDAR FOR THE UK

This calendar shows the general pattern of pollen release in the UK. The exact timing and severity of pollen seasons will vary from year to year depending on the weather, and also regionally depending on geographical location.

Generalised pollen calendar chart showing pollen seasons and peak periods across the months Jan–Sep for the following plants:

Plant (Genus)	Pollen season	Peak period
Hazel (Corylus)	Jan–Apr	Feb
Yew (Taxus)	Feb–Apr	Feb
Elm (Ulmus)	Feb–Apr	Mar
Alder (Alnus)	Feb–Apr	Mar
Willow (Salix)	Mar–May	Mar
Ash (Fraxinus)	Apr–May	Apr
Poplar (Populus)	Mar–Apr	Mar
Birch (Betula)	Mar–May	Apr
Oak (Quercus)	Apr–Jun	May
Pine (Pinus)	May–Jun	May
Grass (Gramineae)	May–Sep	Jun–Jul
Oil seed Rape (Brassica napus)	May–Jun	May
Plane (Platanus)	Apr–Jun	May
Dock (Rumex)	May–Jul	Jun
Nettle (Urtica)	May–Sep	Jun–Jul
Lime (Tilia)	Jun–Jul	Jun
Plantain (Plantago)	May–Aug	Jun
Mugwort (Artemisia)	Jul–Sep	Aug

Peak period of pollen release
Pollen season

Information supplied by the National Pollen Research Unit, University College, Worcester.

The graph below shows the generalised variation in the amount of grass pollen in the air at times measured over the period of a day in the UK on warm days during the season of peak release (June and early July).

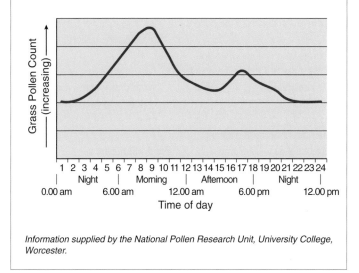

Information supplied by the National Pollen Research Unit, University College, Worcester.

These plants produce huge quantities of pollen. This is because wind pollination is not very efficient. The particles can be carried for long distances, as they are small and dry and therefore light. So this type of pollen is very difficult to avoid. However, there are useful things you can do:

- Identify which pollens cause your allergies by skin-prick testing. You can then find out when to expect trouble from these pollens and start treatment appropriately because each plant flowers at a predictable time each year. Once you know this, you can be prepared.

- Spend as little time out of doors as possible during the pollen season, especially when the pollen count is high. The pollen count will rise on warm, dry, sunny days.

- Try to do your outdoor activities at a time that the pollen count is likely to be lower, for example, early morning or any time after rainfall, which will reduce the pollen count.

- Wear glasses when out of doors, because this will give your eyes some protection from the pollen.

- Change your clothes when you come indoors if the pollen count has been high.

- Do not dry your clothes and bed linen out of doors in summer, because they will become covered in pollen.

- Keep your bedroom window closed during the pollen season.

- If you can, arrange your holiday during the pollen season and go to a country where your trigger pollen is not found. Otherwise, go to the seaside where inshore sea breezes keep the pollen count low.

- If you are allergic to grass pollen, do not cut the grass yourself.

- Some cars now have efficient air filters that trap pollen and make the interior relatively pollen free. Consider choosing one when you next change your car.

- Do your gardening on cold, wet or dull days.

- Choose plants that are insect pollinated, because the pollen from these is much heavier and less likely to cause symptoms.

- Control weeds in the garden, because many of these produce troublesome pollens.

- Avoid things that will make your symptoms worse – such as exposure to smoke, fumes and other forms of air pollution.

Food allergens

Once you have been diagnosed as having an allergy to one or more foodstuffs, face up to your allergy, don't just hope it will go away. The most effective management is to avoid completely the allergen in question (food elimination). You must not eliminate too many food types from your diet at once, otherwise your diet might become deficient in certain essential nutrients. In the case of growing children, no food should be eliminated long term without medical and dietetic advice.

It is important that you do not eliminate foods from your diet unless you have a proven allergy. Many people wrongly blame food allergy for a wide range of symptoms and because of this they limit their choice of food, and therefore their lifestyle, for no real benefit. They may even become malnourished.

Eliminating any foodstuff completely from your diet can be difficult, because it is not always easy to know all the ingredients of packaged and pre-prepared foods. You will need to read food labels very carefully and to learn the different names by which different foodstuffs can be identified. You should read the labels each time you buy a food, as manufacturers sometimes change the ingredients without notice.

All the major supermarket chains provide 'free from' lists, indicating, for example, which foods do not contain egg (see 'Useful addresses', page 94). These are updated regularly and can be very helpful, especially when buying pre-prepared foods. A dietitian can give you helpful advice on 'hidden' sources of different foods.

Some foodstuffs are chemically related to others and so, if you develop an allergy to one, you may also react to another. For example, celery, apple, peanuts and kiwi fruit are all related and their common allergen has been identified. Similarly, bananas, kiwi fruit, papaya, chestnuts and avocados appear to be related, and allergies to all of these can occur in patients who are allergic to latex, although,

as yet, the protein they share is not yet known.

When you are eating out, avoid high-risk restaurants, such as those serving Indian and Eastern dishes, which include a wide range of different ingredients that can be difficult to identify, and in which nuts and peanuts are commonly used. Be direct with the restaurant staff, and ask to speak in person to the chef if you think the waiter is not taking you seriously. Share your problem with your friends so they can help you in choosing appropriate food, and teach them about your symptoms and how to treat them. Be alert and do not ignore any symptom, however mild. It could be the start of a serious reaction. Finally, if you have been prescribed epinephrine, always carry it with you when you go out.

Stinging insects

There are many things you can do to reduce the chances of your being stung by a wasp or bee:

- Use an effective insect repellent when spending time outdoors.

- Wear plain, light-coloured clothes and avoid brightly coloured flower prints and black – these seem to attract insects.

- Never disturb wasp nests or bee hives.

- Do not walk barefoot out of doors.

- Avoid wearing strong perfumes and any cosmetic preparations with a strong fragrance.

- Keep your arms and legs covered.

- Stay away from picnic grounds and the areas around dustbins and litter bins – wasps are particularly attracted by rubbish.

- Keep patios, dustbin areas and barbecues clean.

- Get someone else to mow the lawn.

- Make sure that no bees or wasps are inside your car before you get in.

- If a bee or wasp comes near you, do not attack it, but move slowly and calmly away.

- If an insect lands on you, try to stay calm and leave it alone until it flies away – it will not sting you unless it feels threatened.

DRUG TREATMENTS

It is not possible to avoid all relevant allergens all of the time so, although allergen avoidance should play an important part in the management of your allergies, this approach may need to be combined with the use of appropriate anti-allergy drugs. There are four main groups of drugs:

1 Symptomatic relievers – taken for immediate relief of the symptoms.

2 Antihistamines – which reduce the severity of the allergic reaction by blocking the effects of histamine once it has been released by the inflammatory cells.

3 Anti-inflammatories – which reduce the levels of inflam-mation by preventing the release of the chemicals, including histamine.

4 Leukotriene receptor antagonists – a new class of drug developed specifically for use in allergic diseases. These drugs block the receptor to which leukotrienes (one type of inflammatory chemical) have to attach before they can cause inflammation, so preventing that part of the immune reaction from occurring.

Adrenaline is also used for the treatment of acute/severe allergic reactions (see page 45).

Symptomatic relievers

These drugs should be used to treat

your symptoms only at the time you are experiencing a flare-up.

- **The lungs:** Every person with asthma should carry with them a 'reliever' inhaler, containing a drug that relaxes the airway muscle and dilates the small airways or bronchi (a bronchodilator). It should be in a form that they find easy to use, even when they are breathless and wheezy.

- **The eyes:** A range of eye drops is available that will temporarily reduce the redness, crying and stinging associated with hay fever. These drops contain drugs that constrict the blood vessels on the surface of the eye and reduce the inflammation. However, these drops should not be used for prolonged periods of more than one week. Long-term use will make your condition worse because, when the effects of each dose wear off, your symptoms will reappear worse than before – rebound symptoms. They should also be avoided in people with glaucoma (raised pressure inside the eye), high blood pressure and diabetes.

- **The nose:** Decongestant nose drops or sprays work in the same way as decongestant eye drops, by constricting the blood vessels, but on the lining of the nose. This leads to a decrease in nasal secretions

and relief of nasal obstruction. Although these drugs work rapidly and can be very effective, they should not be used in the long term because they can lead to a worsening of your symptoms. It is far better to protect yourself from your allergic symptoms rather than to treat the end result. You should seek treatment with anti-inflammatories to reduce your inflammatory response and you can avoid the allergen as much as possible.

- **The skin:** Inflamed skin can be very itchy and the regular use of simple emollient creams will not only relieve the itching but will make your skin stronger. These creams do not contain any drugs, but act to smooth the surface of the skin and to increase its degree of hydration by reducing water loss. Both of these actions strengthen your skin by making it thicker and less rough. The creams that your

HELPFUL TIP

If your skin is feeling really itchy, instead of scratching, which will make the itch worse, take a generous handful of emollient cream and rub it gently but firmly into the itchy areas doctor can prescribe for you (some are also available to buy from pharmacies) are more effective than cosmetic moisturiser creams and are less likely to irritate your skin because they contain no perfumes and most are lanolin free.

Antihistamines

Antihistamine drugs act by reducing the ability of histamine to attach to the cell receptor where it exerts its effect. Histamine is one of the most potent inflammatory chemicals released by the body as part of the inflammatory reaction. Histamine can cause airway narrowing, abdominal cramps, sneezing, and itching and watering of the nose and eyes. Antihistamine medications can be supplied as eye drops, nasal sprays and liquid preparations or tablets to take by mouth. Sometimes an antihistamine preparation alone will be enough to prevent your symptoms. However, they are not very good at treating a blocked congested nose caused by hay fever and, for this, an anti-inflammatory preparation (see below) will be needed.

The most common side effect of antihistamines is sedation (drowsiness), and the effect of some of the older antihistamines on your ability to drive may be as serious as the effects of alcohol. These drugs are still used in severe cases of allergy when their sedative effect can be useful in promoting sleep. Chlorpheniramine (Piriton) has probably the greatest sedating effect. It may be useful when you are finding it hard to sleep at night because of your symptoms, but should not be used during the day if you will be driving, cooking or operating machinery. However, some of the new or second-generation drugs are non-sedating – for example, loratadine, acrivastine and astemizole. They are easier to take too, as they are taken once, or at most twice, a day.

Anti-inflammatories

Anti-inflammatory medications reduce the degree of inflammation and so reduce the irritability of the tissues and lessen or even eliminate symptoms. In order to do their job, these medications must be taken regularly, and we generally prefer them to be applied locally to the affected part of the body.

There are two main classes of anti-inflammatory drugs.

• **Sodium cromoglycate and nedocromil:** These preparations are available as eyedrops, nasal sprays, asthma inhalers and for taking by mouth (oral preparations) – although this form is rarely used. It is worth trying these drugs if your symptoms are mild, because they have no side effects whatsoever. However, they are not particularly

ALLERGIC RHINITIS (HAYFEVER): WHICH TREATMENT IS BEST?

	Sneezing/ itch	Watery discharge	Blocked nose	Eye symptoms
Sodium cromoglycate	+	+	−	+
Antihistamines	+++	++	−	+++
Nasal steroids	+++	+++	++	+
Decongestants	−	−	+++	−

− No effect, + limited effectiveness, + + quite effective, + + + very effective.

potent preparations, and may have limited efficacy.

- **Corticosteroids:** The corticosteroid group of drugs is the most useful and effective for the treatment of allergic conditions. They are available in a full range of preparations including skin creams, eye drops, nasal sprays and asthma inhalers, as well as oral preparations, which are used for the treatment of severe or acute symptoms.

Many patients are concerned about using corticosteroid preparations, because they are frightened about possible side effects. First, it is important to understand that corticosteroid medications are not the same as the anabolic steroids sometimes used and abused by body builders and athletes. Second, corticosteroids are usually given topically (locally onto the part of the body that needs treatment), for example, by inhalation for asthma and as creams for eczema. As a result of this, the doses used can be very small, particularly in comparison to the doses that would be needed if taken in tablet form. It is only in high doses and if taken over a prolonged period that corticosteroids will lead to side effects, which may include:

- thin skin

- easy bruising

- thinning of the bones

- underactivity of the adrenal gland – leading to collapse in severe cases

- growth suppression in children.

By using topical preparations from an inhaler, you will be taking between one-fiftieth and one-hundredth of the dose you would have to take orally and you are very unlikely to develop side effects. Unless you have very severe asthma, you will not need to take regular oral steroid preparations, but you may have to take them for a number of days if you have an acute severe attack of your asthma.

Beware, however, if you are using high doses of a steroid inhaler, nose spray or skin cream, or if you are using a combination of these different treatments, because their ability to cause side effects is additive.

If you are taking high doses of any one steroid medication or if you are taking a combination of different steroid medications, you should bring this to the attention of your doctor. He or she will try to reduce the doses you use to the minimum that still provides good treatment of your symptoms. If children are on high doses of steroid treatments, they should be re-evaluated regularly and the doses reduced

wherever possible, and their growth should be carefully monitored.

Leukotriene receptor antagonists

A new class of drug has recently become available for the treatment of asthma – the leukotriene receptor antagonists. These drugs can also be very effective in the treatment of allergic rhinitis and eczema. The two drugs currently available are montelukast and zafirlukast.

For many patients, the best thing about these drugs is that they are taken by mouth in tablet form. These drugs are usually prescribed for people with asthma that is severe enough for them to be taking a steroid inhaler. After a period of treatment you may be able to reduce the dose of your inhaler. If you also have hay fever and eczema, these are likely to improve.

The most common side effect of these drugs is headache, which tends to disappear if you persevere with treatment for a couple of weeks.

Unfortunately, these drugs are not effective in everyone – some people respond well and others not at all. When your doctor starts you on one of these medications, he will probably ask you to keep a record of your symptoms for three to four weeks so that you can both see whether or not you are benefiting.

Epinephrine

Epinephrine is a chemical that occurs naturally in the body, produced by the adrenal gland. Epinephrine has a number of actions, including relaxation of the airways and reversal of the leakiness of the small blood vessels, which may be helpful in the event of a severe allergic reaction.

Epinephrine must be given by injection, usually into a muscle, although in hospital it might be injected directly into a vein. It can be supplied in kits that are easy to use by the patient themselves (see 'Anaphylaxis', page 42). The most popular device, the EpiPen, looks like a pen and can easily be carried with you at all times. Epinephrine works quickly but its effects may wear off after approximately 30 minutes, so a second dose may be required before you reach medical attention. For this reason, you should always carry two devices, and once you have injected epinephrine you should immediately seek medical attention.

IMMUNOTHERAPY

Immunotherapy, also known as desensitisation, is a process by which a patient is rendered less sensitive to an allergen. This is done by giving the patient increasing doses of the substance to which he or she is allergic, starting with extremely small quantities. The allergen is usually given by injection, but may be delivered into the mouth or nose. If this treatment is successful, the numbers of basophils and mast cells are reduced, their sensitivity to allergen is reduced, and the levels of allergen-specific IgE lowered. Immunotherapy should be used only in patients who have an allergy resulting in severe symptoms and which cannot be controlled by conventional drug therapy combined with allergen avoidance. It works best in people who are allergic to only one allergen, although it may work in multiple allergies. The most common conditions treated by immunotherapy include hay fever caused by pollen and severe allergy to bee and wasp stings. Immunotherapy is rarely used for the treatment of asthma. Only one allergen should be treated at any time.

In the UK, a relatively small number of people are treated with immunotherapy because the treatment period is extensive and the risk of serious allergic reactions is high. As a result of the risks, it must only be carried out in specialist allergy centres.

Immunotherapy injections

These are given under the skin (subcutaneously) each week or even twice a week, starting with minute doses. Increasing concentrations of the allergen are used over several months until the highest planned dose is reached. That dose is then repeated once a month to maintain the benefit. The whole course can last several years.

The advantages of this treatment are that in carefully chosen patients this can be a very effective form of therapy and, after completion of the course, the benefits can be long lasting.

The disadvantages are as follows:

- The treatment is time-consuming, as you will need to remain under observation for several hours after each dose and many doses are given, initially as often as twice a week.

- The duration of the course is long, being several years, so it is a major commitment.

- Approximately half of patients suffer a relapse of their symptoms, usually after two to three years.

This treatment can have dangerous side effects. You are being exposed to the allergen responsible for your symptoms, so there is a risk of a severe allergic reaction. This risk is greatest in patients who also have asthma, especially if their asthma is not under good control. Between three and twelve per cent of patients suffer a severe allergic reaction, most of these occurring within 30 minutes of the injection. This is why you are required to remain at the hospital for several hours after each injection.

Very rarely, the allergic reaction can be so severe it is fatal. For this reason, the selection of patients to receive immunotherapy is made very carefully, and the procedure is carried out only by specialists working in specialist centres.

Oral and nasal immunotherapy

In an attempt to reduce the risks of immunotherapy, other routes for giving the doses of allergen have been tried. The oral and nasal routes require higher doses of allergen, are slower to work and carry a greater risk of causing urticaria and angio-oedema. However, the risk of anaphylaxis is lower than with the subcutaneous injections.

Unfortunately, these routes are less effective and the results not as good as with injections. The nasal route seems to provide benefit locally in the nose only, so it is effective only for allergic rhinitis.

WHAT ELSE CAN I DO?

Irritants

Your symptoms should be well controlled if your allergies have been diagnosed correctly, if you have reduced your exposure to the relevant allergen adequately and if you are taking appropriate medication. However, there are other things that you can do to help. If you can avoid exposure to substances likely to cause irritant reactions, you will be less vulnerable to the effects of your allergies.

A wide range of substances can cause irritant reactions of your lungs, nose, eyes and skin, and the most common of these is tobacco smoke. If you currently smoke you should try to give up. If you are a non-smoker, you should reduce as much as possible your exposure to other people's cigarette smoke. Babies and small children should never be allowed to breathe in cigarette smoke.

Raised levels of air pollutants – for example, car exhaust fumes, ozone, cigarette smoke, formaldehyde and nitrous oxide – can also make your allergy symptoms worse. As we spend most of our time indoors it makes sense to keep our home environment as free as possible from smoke and fumes. Keep your house well ventilated, especially the rooms that contain a gas burner of any kind. At work, make sure that your employer protects you from inhaling any dusts or fumes. Outdoors, avoid walking along busy roads where you will be exposed to high levels of car exhaust fumes and dust, if you can.

Identification jewellery

If you or your child has a severe allergy, you may find it reassuring to wear a piece of medical identification jewellery which carries details of your medical problem as well as your personal details and your doctor's name and telephone number. These can be provided by a number of different companies, each of which offers a different service. Details of how to contact Medic-Alert, SOS Talisman and Golden Key can be found under 'Useful addresses' (page 94). Medic-Alert, a charity established in 1965, maintains an up-to-date computerised database of its members' medical conditions and they make this available to the emergency services.

Complementary therapies

There is a wide range of different treatments offered by a variety of practitioners. I think it is important to draw the distinction between *alternative* therapies, which aim to replace the treatments offered by the medical profession, and *complementary* therapies, which are intended for use alongside conventional treatments. As the effects of severe allergy can be very unpleasant and even life threatening, it is important that you do not

What training have you had?

What are your qualifications?

How much experience do you have?

Are you registered with a recognised organisation?

What will the treatment involve?

Is this the best treatment for me?

What benefits can I expect?

Will you tell my GP about this treatment?

Are you happy for me to continue my normal medications?

How many sessions do you recommend?

How much will this cost?

suddenly stop the medications prescribed for you by your doctor. If an alternative therapist tells you that his or her treatments will not work unless you give up your other medications, speak to your doctor first. In my opinion, other therapies work best when used in conjunction with conventional medicine.

Very little is known about how complementary therapies work, but, if you find one that works for you and you can afford the treatment, then I would encourage you to use it. However, complementary therapies should never be relied on in the case of a sudden acute allergic reaction, when conventional medicines will offer you the most effective solutions. It is worth bearing in mind that many complementary therapists have no formal medical training and might not have the experience or the knowledge to diagnose and treat your medical problems properly. Other diseases can sometimes mimic the symptoms of allergy, and may be misdiagnosed by complementary therapists.

Complementary therapies are often regarded as a low-risk option, but dangerous side effects can occur and, at worst, they could actually kill you. The Chinese herbal medicine *Aristolochia* has caused kidney failure in a number of patients and was banned in 1999. In

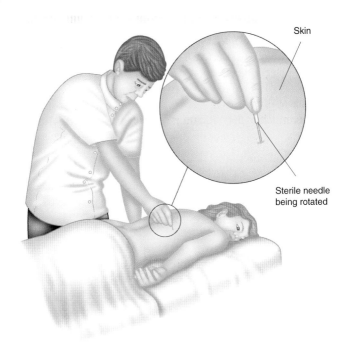

Skin

Sterile needle being rotated

Acupuncture is a method of pain relief that involves insertion of fine sterile needles into specific points on the body. The needles may then be rotated to produce stimulation.

1998, 12 patients contracted hepatitis B, which is potentially fatal, in London from a therapy called autohaemotherapy.

In the UK there are 40,000 complementary therapists and they now outnumber registered GPs (31,000). Yet complementary therapists are largely unregulated, and registration with a professional body is not compulsory. If you are thinking of seeking help from a complementary therapist, it is worth ensuring that they are suitably qualified and regulated. You can contact the Department of Health (see 'Useful addresses', page 96) and ask if they will give you the names of recommended practitioners in your area. Your GP might also be able to help you with this. You can also contact the relevant professional body, such as the British Acupuncture Council (see 'Useful addresses', page 100). See also *Understanding Complementary Medicine*, another book in the Family Doctor series.

BRIEF GUIDE TO COMPLEMENTARY MEDICINE

- **Acupuncture:** Acupuncture is an ancient Chinese medical practice. Diagnosis is based on an assessment of the patient's mood, character and life situation. Treatment aims to improve the flow of energy through clearly defined channels in the body, clearing blockages to this flow, which result in illness.

This is done by the insertion of very fine steel needles into specific points along the channels of energy flow. The needles are left in place for between 5 and 30 minutes. Although acupuncture is sometimes recommended for asthma and hay fever, the treatments need to be very frequent and, as yet, there is no scientific proof that it offers any benefit for these conditions.

- **Homoeopathy:** The practice of homoeopathy is based on the theory that 'like cures like'. Minute quantities of the substance believed to mimic the symptoms of disease are given to treat that disease. The remedies are taken by mouth.

The results of homoeopathy can be slow and initially symptoms may become worse. However, the remedies are felt to be safe because they contain such tiny quantities of the substance used. Although homoeopathy is recommended for the treatment of all allergic diseases by its practitioners, it is only in hay

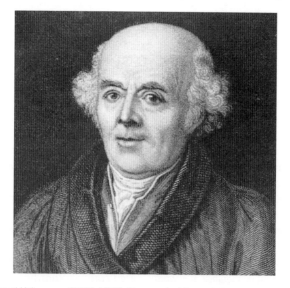

Dr Samuel Hahnemann (1755–1843), German physician and pioneer of homoeopathy.

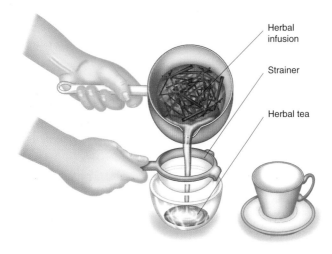

Herbal medicine involves the use of plant extracts to treat illness. The remedy is often prepared as a 'tea' to drink.

fever that homoeopathy seems to offer a benefit detectable by scientific studies.

• **Enzyme-potentiated desensitisation:** In this treatment a very small dose of the allergen or a number of different relevant allergens is mixed with an enzyme (beta-glucuronidase) and the mixture injected under the skin. A single dose is said to give lasting benefit, and its supporters believe that it is effective in many different allergic diseases.

However, at the moment there is very little evidence to prove this and more studies are needed. Severe adverse reactions to this treatment can occur and it should

only be performed in a place where such reactions can be quickly and properly treated and resuscitation given if needed, for example, a specialised allergy clinic or a sizeable hospital.

• **Herbal medicine:** Herbal medicines made from the leaves, flowers, bark or roots of plants have been used for thousands of years. In some parts of the world it is the only form of medicine used. Western herbalists prescribe a combination of different herbal remedies specific to an individual's problem. In addition, Chinese herbal therapies have gained in popularity and have been found to be very effective in eczema. However, some products have been found to be contaminated with other substances such as steroid preparations, and others have led to serious complications such as liver damage. Only seek treatment from a reputable therapist (see 'Useful Addresses', page 100).

KEY POINTS

✓ We cannot yet cure allergies

✓ Most people's symptoms can be well controlled using a combination of drug treatment and allergen avoidance

✓ Whatever the allergen to which you are allergic, there are many practical ways in which you can reduce your exposure to it

✓ The most common allergy in the UK is to the house-dust mite

✓ The indoor environment is the most important as we spend about 90 per cent of our time indoors

✓ Learn all about your drug treatment, including how and when to use it, so that you may use it effectively

✓ Immunotherapy is used only in people whose allergy symptoms are severe and in whom drug treatment and allergen avoidance are not effective

✓ A wide range of complementary therapies is available

✓ Choose your complementary therapist with care

Living with allergies

SCHOOL

If your child has an allergic condition, you may be anxious about how well the school is able to cope. It may help to remember that as many as one in three of the children in the school will have some type of allergic condition and the teachers will have considerable experience in dealing with related problems. However, it is only sensible to make sure that the school has all the information that may be relevant to your child and his or her medical problem. Include the following information:

- The condition your child has

- The things your child is allergic to

- The names and doses of the medications your child takes regularly

- The names and doses of the medications your child will need to take at school on a regular basis

- The names and doses of the medications your child might need to take in the event of an allergic reaction

- A treatment plan of exactly what to do if your child develops an allergic reaction

- Details of the triggers known to make your child's condition worse

- The name and telephone number of your general practitioner

- Telephone numbers where you, your partner and other nominated adults can be contacted in an emergency.

Every school receives instructions from the Department for Education and Skills (DfES), in conjunction with the local education authority, on putting an asthma policy in place, covering details such as the storage and administration of children's asthma inhalers in school. If your child has other allergies, you might find it helpful to give the school relevant information such as that produced by Allergy UK or the Anaphylaxis Campaign (see 'Useful addresses', page 95).

If your child has a severe allergic problem, it is important to spend some time with the relevant members of staff to discuss your child's needs. In the UK, all children, including those with special medical needs, have a right to full education in state schools, and their teachers must, within reason, take responsibility for the child's medical needs while they are at school. The DfES and the Department of Health have issued joint guidelines on supporting pupils with medical needs in school. Copies can be obtained from the DfES (see 'Useful addresses', page 96).

Food

Food in school can be an issue for children with food allergies. It should still be possible for children with food allergies to eat school meals, but they will need special supervision by a member of staff to ensure that they make appropriate choices. It may be easier to provide your child with a packed lunch. Many schools now have a no-sharing policy to ensure that children eat only the food provided for them. Make sure that your child will have access to their medications at all times in case they accidentally eat the wrong food.

Exercise and sport

Exercise and sport can present difficulties to many children with allergic problems. Exercise can make asthma worse. Outdoor sports may expose children to high levels of pollen that could make asthma, hay fever or eczema worse. Although swimming is a form of exercise well tolerated by children with asthma, it can make eczema much worse. There are ways of getting round these problems (see 'Useful publications, page 102) so that all children are able to join in with all school activities including sport.

Hay fever

Some parents worry that their child's hay fever may affect their performance in examinations, which generally take place during the pollen season. The following may be helpful:

- Start appropriate preventive

medications before the hay fever season commences. It is harder to gain control of symptoms once they have started than it is to prevent them.

- Your child may need to use more than one medication. Often the combination of an antihistamine, a nasal spay and eye drops works best.

- Make sure that your child takes medications regularly.

- Follow the advice on pollen avoidance (see 'Treatment of allergic disease', page 62).

- If your child is sitting examinations and is troubled by hay fever, ask the school or college to inform the examining board.

HOLIDAYS AND TRAVEL

Some people, especially those with severe allergic problems, never go away on holiday because of their fear of what may happen in an unknown environment. It is a great shame because, with the right information and some forward planning, a holiday can be a very enjoyable experience regardless of the allergy.

It is possible to remove or at least minimise many potential hazards by maintaining control over the important aspects of your life while you are on holiday. For example, if you have a severe food allergy, you could choose to stay in self-catering accommodation. If you have hay fever, you might choose to visit the southern hemisphere where not only will the season differ from that at home but also the local pollens will differ. Alternatively you might consider a seaside holiday because the pollen count is generally lower on the coast. If you have asthma, you may be able to take appropriate rescue medications with you so that, with careful instructions from your doctor, you could treat any exacerbation early.

Do remember to take sufficient supplies of your medication to last throughout the holiday with you, and always carry your medications in your hand luggage just in case your main luggage goes astray. Other points to remember are:

- Choose a destination that in your experience is least likely to trigger your allergy.

- If you have any special requirements, such as a special diet or feather-free bedding, ask your holiday company to supply these well in advance and ask for confirmation in writing.

- Make sure you have adequate medical insurance and do tell your insurer about your medical problem.

GENERAL ADVICE FOR PARENTS OF CHILDREN WITH ALLERGIES

Remember the following:

- Make sure that your child takes his or her preventive medications regularly.

- Make sure children have access to their reliever medications at all times while in school.

- If your child has asthma and exercise is a problem, advise taking two puffs of their reliever inhaler at least 15 minutes before exercise.

- If your child has eczema, make sure she or he wears natural fibres (for example, cotton) next to the skin and avoid wool, which can irritate the skin.

- If your child has eczema, make sure she or he can shower thoroughly after swimming to remove the chemicals and, if needed, re-apply their emollient cream.

- If your child has a food allergy, make sure the school is well informed of this. Ensure that the school dining room has a no-sharing policy. Ask the school to warn you in advance of what ingredients will be used in domestic science (cookery) lessons and ask whether the relevant food stuffs might be avoided.

- Find out whether the school has any pets or other animals on the premises. If they do and your child is allergic to them, ask if you may visit the school to discuss how your child might avoid exposure to the allergen.

- If your child has a **severe** food allergy, make sure the school and the child's classmates are well aware of this, and request that all of the children be made to wash their hands and faces thoroughly after eating so that food allergens are not spread around by touch after meals.

- If you are going to a European Union country, take with you form E111, available from any post office – you can use it to get free medical care.

- Take with you a written action plan covering what you would do if you have an exacerbation while on holiday.

- Check the expiry dates of your medications.

- If you have been prescribed an epinephrine device, take extra supplies with you in case you need to use them more than once. It will be difficult to organise replacements abroad.

- Protect your epinephrine device from extremes of temperature (don't leave it in the car), and discard it if the epinephrine becomes discoloured.

- If you have a severe food allergy, contact the airline in advance, stating the type and severity of your allergy. If you are allergic to peanuts, ask whether the flight is peanut free (many airlines now ban peanuts).

- As soon as you arrive, locate the nearest telephone and find out the telephone numbers of the nearest doctor, ambulance service and hospital accident and emergency department.

- Remember that the telephone number for the emergency services (999 in the UK) varies from country to country.

- Teach your travelling companions what to do if you have an acute severe allergic reaction.

- Take with you a letter from your doctor explaining what your medication is and confirming that it is for your own personal use. This should avoid any problems at Customs and Excise inspections.

- If you do not speak the language of the country you are visiting, Allergy UK and the Anaphylaxis Campaign (see 'Useful addresses', page 95) can provide you with a range of cards carrying translations of important messages.

Bon voyage!

FINANCE

Having an allergic condition can be costly, not only because of all those prescription costs but also because of the cost of special diets, non-allergic and protective bedding, and other special equipment that you might need. If you are not exempt from paying prescription charges, a pre-payment certificate may reduce the cost. Currently, if you require more than five items in a four-month period, pre-payment works out cheaper, because, after paying the flat fee, all prescriptions are free, no matter how many you need. To obtain a pre-payment certificate contact your local health authority or ask at your pharmacy. Some medications are cheaper to buy over the counter from your pharmacist than paying a prescription charge. Your pharmacist can advise you on this. He or she can also provide you with a leaflet called *Are*

you entitled to help with health costs?

If you need a special diet, some foodstuffs can be prescribed by your GP. Most people on special diets receive no financial help, but your modified diet need not be expensive. Allergy UK and the Anaphylaxis Campaign (see 'Useful addresses', page 95) are good sources of information about special cookbooks. All of the major supermarkets provide 'free from' lists which can be very helpful in identifying foods that are safe for you to eat (see 'Useful addresses', page 94).

KEY POINTS

✓ With the right information and support, your children's schools will be able to cope with all issues relating to their allergic conditions

✓ Even children with severe allergies should be able to join in most activities at school

✓ With careful forward planning, a holiday can be a very enjoyable experience even if you have severe allergies

✓ Before you go on holiday, make sure you have adequate medical insurance and, for the EU, complete form E111, available from any post office

✓ If you are not exempt from paying prescription charges, a pre-payment certificate may reduce the cost

The future

Allergic diseases are becoming more common, and at present doctors can only treat these conditions, not cure them. However, we are learning all the time, and new and important discoveries are being made every year.

We have learned a great deal recently about the factors that increase our children's chances of developing allergic diseases, and the result of this is that we can now develop prevention methods. Some of these are very simple, for example, ensuring that babies and young children are NEVER exposed to tobacco smoke. Some are more complex, for example, programmes to reduce the levels of exposure in infancy to a number of different allergens including foods and the house-dust mite. If you are interested in taking part in this type of medical research, one of the large research charities such as Allergy UK may be able to put you in contact with a local research group.

Major advances have been made in learning about the genetics of allergy. Our genetic material is found on our chromosomes. Chromosomes are made of DNA and carry our genes – the units of genetic material that determine the characteristics we inherit from our parents. Scientists are currently trying to identify the genes responsible for the development of different allergic conditions. Once these genes are known, it may be possible to develop new drugs designed specifically to target certain aspects of the disease. In the longer term, it may be possible to repair faulty genes and provide a cure.

Work is also going on to investigate the possibility of immunising against allergy. Although this seems a very attractive option, we do not know yet whether a vaccine would be effective and, just as importantly, whether it would be safe.

While we are waiting for these dreams to become reality, we can still take advantage of the new drugs that have been developed over the past few years. The newer antihistamines are virtually non-sedating, more effective and have the advantage of a once-a-day dosage schedule. The leukotriene receptor antagonists are showing great promise for selected patients, and patients with asthma are very enthusiastic about these drugs as they are taken by mouth.

Finally, as you learn more about the way in which allergic reactions happen, what the common trigger factors for allergy are and how to avoid them, you will be able to manage your symptoms effectively and so improve the quality of your life and the lives of your loved ones. I hope this book has succeeded in helping you achieve that.

Useful addresses

GENERAL

Action Against Allergy
PO Box 278
Twickenham
Middx TW1 4QQ
Tel: 020 8892 2711
Fax: 020 8892 4950
Email: AAA@actionagainstallergy.
freeserve.co.uk
Website:
www.actionagainstallergy.co.uk

A support charity, providing information (including holiday and accommodation), suppliers' lists and
newsletter advice on specialist re-
ferral. Send an s.a.e. for information.

Action on Smoking and Health (ASH)
102 Clifton Street
London EC2A 4HW
Tel: 020 7739 5902
Fax: 020 7613 0531
Email: enquiries@ash.org.uk
Website: www.ash.org.uk

A national organisation with
branches throughout the UK.
Campaigns on anti-smoking policies
offering free information on website
or for sale from HQ. Catalogue on
request.

Allerayde Ltd
Freepost NG2687
1B Enterprise Park
Brunel Drive
Newark
Notts NG24 2DZ
Tel: 01636 613609
Fax: 01636 612161
Email: info@allerayde.co.uk
Website: www.allerayde.co.uk

Distributor of dustproof bedding
and other products such as sleeping
suits for children and adults. Mail
order only; catalogue on request.

AllergyFree Direct Ltd
Conna-Mara
Maer Down Road
Crooklets Beach
Bude
Cornwall EX23 8NG
Tel/fax: 01288 356396
Email: comments@allergyfreedirect.com

Mail order specialist for foods free from wheat, gluten, milk and eggs; vegan and vegetarian foods also available. The website is easy to navigate with the categories clearly labelled and giving the ingredients used for each product. It also contains a glossary.

Allergy UK (formerly British Allergy Foundation)
Deepdene House
30 Bellegrove Road
Welling
Kent DA16 3PY
Tel: 020 8303 8525
Helpline: 020 8303 8583 (9am–9pm Mon–Fri, 10am–1pm Sat and Sun)
Email: info@allergyuk.org
Website: www.allergyuk.org

Encompasses all types of allergies, food and chemical sensitivities, and offers information, quarterly newsletter and support network; translation cards available to members for travel abroad. Annual subscription 2004: £15.

Anaphylaxis Campaign
PO Box 275
Farnborough
Hampshire GU14 6SX
Tel: 01252 373793
Fax: 01252 377140
Helpline: 01252 542029
Email: info@anaphylaxis.org.uk
Website: www.anaphylaxis.org.uk

Campaigns for better awareness of life-threatening allergic reactions from food and other allergies to bee and wasp stings. Produces a wide range of educational news sheets and has extensive support network.

Asda
Customer Services Department
Asda House
Great Wilson Street
Leeds LS11 5AD
Tel: 0113 243 5434
Fax: 0113 241 7732
Helpline: 0500 100055
Minicom: 0800 068 3003
Website: www.asda.co.uk

'Free from' booklets available on request and on website.

Benefits Enquiry Line
Tel: 0800 882200
N. Ireland: 0800 220674
Minicom: 0800 243355

Government agency giving information and advice on sickness and disability benefits for people with disabilities and their carers.

Boots Customer Services
1 Thane Road
Nottingham NG2 3AA
Tel: 0115 950 6111
Helpline: 0845 070 8090
Website: www.boots.com

Will provide, on request, 'free from' lists on their own-brand products (not available on website). Also produces infant formulas.

British Society for Allergy and Clinical Immunology (BSACI)
17 Doughty Street
London WC1N 2PL
Tel: 020 7404 0278
Fax: 020 7404 0280
Email: info@bsaci.org
Website: www.bsaci.org

Produces a regularly updated list of NHS allergy clinics throughout the country.

Coeliac UK (formerly Coeliac Society of the UK)
PO Box 220
High Wycombe
Buckinghamshire HP11 2HY
Tel: 01494 437278
Fax: 01494 474349
Helpline: 0870 444 8804
Email: admin@coeliac.co.uk
Website: www.coeliac.co.uk

Provides information and support for people medically diagnosed with coeliac disease or dermatitis herpetiformis.

Co-op
Customer Services
CWS Ltd
PO Box 53
New Century House
Manchester M60 4ES
Tel: 0161 834 1212
Helpline: 0800 068 6727
Minicom: 0800 0684 244
Email: customerrelations@co-op.co.uk
Website: www.co-op.co.uk

Will provide, on request, 'free from' lists free of charge for their own-brand products.

Cosmetic Toiletry & Perfumery Association (CTPA) Ltd
Josaron House
5–7 John Princes Street
London W1G 0JN
Tel: 020 7491 8891
Fax: 020 7493 8061
Email: info@ctpa.org.uk
Website: www.ctpa.org.uk

Association for professionals, providing details of cosmetic ingredients only to its members, not the general public.

Department of Education and Skills (DfES)
PO Box 5050
Sherwood Park
Annesley
Nottinghamshire NG15 0DJ
Helpline: 0870 002288
Publications: 0845 602 2260
Email: dfes@prolog.uk.com
Website: www.dfes.gov.uk

Government information centre which refers callers to different departments as appropriate. Publishes several reports including *Supporting Pupils with Medical Needs* and *Supporting Pupils with Medical Needs in Schools*.

Department for Environment, Food and Rural Affairs (DEFRA) (formerly MAFF)
17 Smith Square
London SW1P 3JR
Helpline: 0845 933 5577
Email: helpline@defra.gsi.gov.uk
Website: www.defra.gov.uk

Implements Government policies and publishes information about environmental, rural and farming matters and food production. Enquiries about allergies now dealt with by the Food Standards Agency (see below).

Department of Health
PO Box 77
London SE1 6XH

Tel: 020 7210 4850
Fax: 01623 724524
Helpline: 0800 555777 (health literature line)
Textline: 01623 756236
Website: www.doh.gov.uk

Produces and distributes literature about public health. Enquiries about allergies now dealt with by the Food Standards Agency (see below).

Food Standards Agency
Aviation House
125 Kingsway
London WC2B 6NH
Tel: 020 7276 8000
Publications: 0845 606 0667

For queries about specific sensitivities or allergies:

Additives: 020 7276 8570
Allergies and intolerances: 020 7276 8516
Chemical safety: 020 7276 8527
Contaminants: 020 7276 8713
Novel foods: 020 7276 8595

Foresight
28 The Paddock
Godalming
Surrey GU7 1XD
Tel: 01483 427839
Fax: 01483 427668
Website: www.foresight-preconception.org.uk

Gives advice and counselling on preconceptual care.

Golden Key
1 Hare Street
Sheerness

Kent ME12 1AH
Tel: 01795 663403
Fax: 01795 661356

Provides engraving service for SOS identification jewellery. Individual service available by mail order.

Health and Safety Executive
Information Services
Caerphilly Business Park
Cardiff CF83 3GG
Helpline: 0870 154 5500 (8am–6pm Mon–Fri)
Textphone: 029 3080 8537
Fax: 02920 859 260
Email: hseinformationservices@natbrit.com
Website: www.hse.gov.uk

Offers information and advice about health and safety regulations in the workplace and their implementation.

Holiday Care
7th Floor, Sunley House
4 Bedford Park
Croydon CR0 2AP
Tel: 0845 124 9971
Fax: 0845 124 9972
Minicom: 0845 124 9976
Email: info@holidaycare.org
Website: www.holidaycare.org.uk

Provides holiday advice on venues and tour operators for people with special needs, including transport, insurance, oxygen supplies, etc. in the UK and abroad. Publishes information sheets on overseas destinations. Offers professional consultancy service to the tourism industry.

Institute of Translation and Interpreting

Fortuna House
South Fifth Street
Milton Keynes MK9 2EU
Tel: 01908 325250
Fax: 01908 325259
Email: info@iti.org.uk
Website: www.iti.org.uk

Institute for translators and interpreters; most languages covered.

Marks and Spencer

Customer Services
Chester Business Park
Wrexham Road
Chester CH4 9GA
Tel: 0845 302 1234
Fax: 0845 303 0170
Email: retailcustomerservices@marks-and-spencer.com
Website: www.marksandspencer.com

Will provide, on request, information on own-brand foods that are suitable for special diets (diabetes not included).

MedicAlert

1 Bridge Wharf
Caledonian Road
London N1 9UU
Tel: 020 7833 3034
Fax: 020 7278 0647
Email: info@medicalert.org.uk
Website: www.medicalert.org.uk

Provides emergency identification with body-worn jewellery for people with hidden medical conditions and allergies; 24-hour emergency telephone which accepts reverse charge calls; can access personal details from anywhere in the world in over 100 languages.

National Asthma Campaign

Providence House
Providence Place
London N1 0NT
Tel: 020 7226 2260
Fax: 020 7704 0740
Helpline: 08457 010203 (9am–5pm weekdays)
Email: asthmanurse.org.uk
Website: www.asthma.org.uk

Publications about asthma and its management and helpline run by team of asthma nurse specialists.

National Eczema Society

Hill House
Highgate Hill
London N19 5NA
Tel: 020 7281 3553
Fax: 020 7281 6395
Helpline: 0870 241 3604 (Mon–Fri 11am–4pm); textphone also on this number
Website: www.eczema.org

Provides information, newsletter and helpline for people with eczema and for parents of children with eczema. Support network.

National Pollen Research Unit

University College Worcester
Worcester WR2 6AJ
Tel: 01905 855000
Email: pollen@worc.ac.uk
Website: www.worc.ac.uk

This website offers pollen forecasts and links to other allergy-related organisations.

National Institute for Clinical Excellence (NICE)
MidCity Place
71 High Holborn
London WC1V 6NA
Tel: 020 7067 5800
Fax: 020 7067 5801
Email: nice@nice.nhs.uk
Website: www.nice.org.uk

Provides guidance on treatments and care for people using the NHS in England and Wales. Patient information leaflets are available for each piece of guidance issued.

Safeway Nutrition Advice Service
Safeway Stores plc
6 Millington Road
Hayes
Middlesex UB3 4AY
Tel: 020 8848 8744
Email: nutrition@safeway.co.uk
Website: www.safeway.co.uk

Will provide, on request, information on own-brand products that are suitable for special diets. (This information is also available on the actual product labels.)

Sainsbury's Supermarkets Ltd
Customer Services
33 Holborn
London EC1N 2HT
Helpline: 0800 636262
Website: www.sainsbury.co.uk

'Free from' lists for various special diets available on request.

Somerfield Stores Ltd
Customer Services
Somerfield House

Whitchurch Lane
Bristol BS14 0TJ
Tel: 0117 935 9359
Helpline: 0117 935 6669
Website: www.somerfield.co.uk

'Free from' lists for various special diets available on request.

SOS Talisman Ltd
Talman Ltd
21 Grays Corner
Ley Street
Ilford, Essex IG2 7RQ
Tel: 020 8554 5579
Fax: 020 8554 1090

Suppliers of pendants/bracelets that contain information on the wearer's allergies.

Tesco
Customer Services
Freepost SCO2298
Baird Avenue
Dundee DD1 1YP
Helpline: 0800 505555
Fax: 01382 822230
Email: customer.service@tesco.co.uk
Website: www.tesco.com

'Free from' lists for various special diets available on request.

UCB Institute of Allergy
UCB House
3 George Street
Watford
Herts WD18 8UH
Tel: 01923 211811
Fax: 01923 229002
Email: instituteofallergy.uk@ucb-group.com
Website:
www.theucbinstituteofallergy.com

Information and action, through research and advice, and informing both health professionals and the public on pertinent issues.

Waitrose
Nutritional Advice Centre, Waitrose
Southern Industrial Area
Bracknell
Berks RG12 8YA
Tel: 01344 824975
Fax: 01344 824990
Email: customer_service@waitrose.co.uk
Website: www.waitrose.com

'Free from' lists for various special diets available on request.

COMPLEMENTARY MEDICINE

British Acupuncture Association
22 Hockley Road
Rayleigh
Essex M33 4RA
Tel: 01268 742534
Fax: 01268 772142

British Acupuncture Council
63 Jeddo Road
London W12 9HQ
Tel: 020 8735 0400
Fax: 020 8735 0404
Email: info@acupuncture.org.uk
Website: www.acupuncture.org.uk

Professional body offering lists of qualified acupuncture therapists.

British Homeopathic Association
Hahnemann House
20 Park Street West
Luton LU1 3BE
Tel: 08704 443 950
Fax: 08704 443 960

Email: info@trusthomeopathy.org
Website: www.trusthomeopathy.org

Professional body offering lists of qualified homoeopathic practitioners.

British Medical Acupuncture Society
BMAS House
3 Winnington Court
Northwich
Cheshire CW8 1AQ
Tel: 01606 786782
Fax: 01606 786783
Email: admin@medical-acupuncture.org.uk
Website: www.medical-acupuncture.co.uk

Professional body offering training in acupuncture to doctors and lists of accredited practitioners in local areas.

General Chiropractic Council
44 Wicklow Street
London WC1X 9HL
Tel: 020 7713 5155
Fax: 020 7713 5844
Helpline: 0845 601 1796
Email: enquiries@gcc-uk.org
Website: www.gcc-uk.org

Professional body for chiropractors which can provide details of registered practitioners in your area.

General Osteopathic Council
Osteopathy House
176 Tower Bridge Road
London SE1 3LU
Tel: 020 7357 6655
Fax: 020 7357 0011
Email: info@osteopathy.org.uk
Website: www.osteopathy.org.uk

Regulatory body which offers information about osteopathy to the public and lists of accredited osteopaths in local areas.

Institute of Complementary Medicine
PO Box 194
London SE16 7QZ
Tel: 020 7237 5165
Fax: 020 7237 5175
Email: icm@icmedicine.co.uk
Website: www.icmedicine.co.uk

A registered charity formed as umbrella for complementary medicine groups. Recommends approved training courses and has register of accredited British practitioners. For information please send an s.a.e. with two 1st class stamps.

International Federation of Reflexologists
76–78 Edridge Road
Croydon
Surrey CR0 1EF
Tel: 020 8645 9134
Fax: 020 8649 9291

Professional body representing reflexologists internationally.

National Institute of Medical Herbalists
56 Longbrook Street
Exeter EX4 6AH
Tel: 01392 426022
Fax: 01392 498963
Email: nimh@ukexeter.freeserve.co.uk
Website: www.nimh.org.uk

Professional body representing qualified, practising medical herbalists. Offers list of accredited medical herbalists in your area. Please send an s.a.e.

Register of Chinese Herbal Medicine
Office 5, Ferndale Business Centre
1 Exeter Street
Norwich NR2 4QB
Tel: 01603 623994
Fax: 01603 667557
Email: herbmed@rchm.co.uk
Website: www.rchm.co.uk

Regulatory body holding register of practitioners in the UK appropriately trained in Chinese herbal medicine. For list of qualified members, an s.a.e. is requested.

MEDICAL EQUIPMENT

Clement Clarke International Ltd
Edinburgh Way
Harlow
Essex CM20 2TT
Tel: 01279 414969
Fax: 01279 456304
Website: www.clement-clarke.com

Suppliers of peak flowmeters, spacers and nebulisers.

Dunlopillo and Slumberland
Salmon Fields
Ryton
Oldham OL2 6SB
Tel: 0161 628 2898
Fax: 0161 628 7680
Email: enquiries@dunlopillo.co.uk
Website: www.dunlopillo.co.uk

Manufacturers of latex foam mattresses, pillows and beds.

Medivac Healthcare Ltd
Freepost LON12778
London NW11 6YR
Tel: 0845 130 6969
Fax: 0845 130 6868
Helpline: 0845 130 6164
Email: medivacuk@aol.com
Website: www.medivac.co.uk

Supplies specialised vacuum cleaners, bedding, air filters, etc. for those with asthma, eczema, rhinitis, etc.

Profile Therapeutics plc (formerly Medic-Aid Ltd)
Heath Place
Bognor Regis
West Sussex PO22 9SL
Tel: 0870 770 2000
Fax: 0870 770 2001
Email: info@profiletherapeutics.com
Website: www.profilehs.com

Supplies nebulisers, compressors, facemasks and spacer devices.

Vitalograph Ltd
Maids Moreton House
Maids Moreton
Buckingham MK18 1SW
Tel: 01280 827110
Fax: 01280 823302
Email: sales@vitalograph.co.uk
Website: www.vitalograph.co.uk

Supplies spirometers and emergency resuscitation equipment as well as training on their use.

Vorwerk (UK) Ltd
Vorwerk House
Ashville Way
Wokingham
Berks RG41 2PL
Tel: 0118 989 6522

Fax: 0118 977 2888
Website: www.vorwerk.co.uk

Manufactures and supplies vacuum cleaners.

FURTHER WEBSITE ADDRESSES

www.allallergy.net
Big website giving list of allergy-related websites.

www.allergies.about.com
All about allergies, in user-friendly language.

www.allerex.ca
All about how to use the EpiPen.

www.amazon.com
On-line bookshop.

www.boots.com (formerly Boots.co.uk)
Information on products including those for allergy.

www.foodallergy.org
Website of the Food Allergy and Anaphylaxis Network (a non-profit-making organisation in the USA)

www.peanutallergy.com
American site on peanut allergy.

USEFUL PUBLICATIONS

In addition to the publications listed here, the various allergy associations, organisations and self-help groups publish a wide range of magazines, booklets, leaflets and fact sheets. Contact them at the addresses given for an up-to-date publications list.

General

Joanne Clough (1998) *Allergies at Your Fingertips*. London: Class Publishing.

Myron Lipkowitz (1994) *Allergies A–Z*. Facts on File.

Anne Woodham (1994) *HEA Guide to Complementary Medicine and Therapies*. London: Health Education Authority.

M. Eric Gershwin (1992) *Living Allergy Free*. London: Humana Press.

Asthma

Mark Levy, Sean Hilton and Greta Barnes (1997) *Asthma at Your Fingertips*, 2nd edn. London: Class Publishing.

Jenny Lewis with the National Asthma Campaign (1996) *The Asthma Handbook*. London: Vermilion.

John Donaldson (1994) *Living with Asthma and Hayfever*, revised edn. Harmondsworth: Penguin.

If you have asthma because of your work, NI237, issued by the Department of Social Security and available on request from your local Social Security offices, may be helpful.

Skin allergies

David J. Atherton (1995) *Eczema in Childhood – the Facts*, revised edn. Oxford: Oxford University Press.

Jenny Lewis with the National Eczema Society (1994) *The Eczema Handbook*. London: Vermilion.

Hay fever

Deryk Williams, Anna Williams and Laura Croker (1997) *Living with Asthma and Hayfever*. London: Piatkus Books.

Education

Your Guide to the NHS (formerly the Patient's Charter), published by the Department of Health (single copies available free of charge by calling 0800 555777).

Special Educational Needs – A guide for parents, published by the Department for Education and Skills (single copies available free from the DfES Publications Centre by calling 0845 602 2260).

Supporting Pupils with Medical Needs in Schools, published by the Department for Education and Skills (single copies available free from the DfES Publications Centre by calling 0845 602 2260).

Travel
Health Advice for Travellers, published by the Department of Health (single copies available free of charge by calling 0800 555777).

THE INTERNET AS A SOURCE OF FURTHER INFORMATION

After reading this book, you may feel that you would like further information on the subject. One source is the internet and there are a great many websites with useful information about medical disorders, related charities and support groups. Some websites, however, have unhelpful and inaccurate information. Many are sponsored by commercial organisations or raise revenue by advertising, but nevertheless aim to provide impartial and trustworthy health information. Others may be reputable but you should be aware that they may be biased in their recommendations. Remember that treatment advertised on international websites may not be available in the UK.

Unless you know the address of the specific website that you want to visit (for example, familydoctor. co.uk), you may find the following guidelines helpful when searching the internet.

There are several different sorts of websites that you can use to look for information, the main ones being search engines, directories and portals.

Search engines and directories
There are many search engines and directories that all use different algorithms (procedures for computation) to return different results when you do a search. Search engines use computer programs called spiders, which crawl the web on a daily basis to search individual pages within a site and then queue them ready for listing in their database.

Directories, however, consider a site as a whole and use the description and information that was provided with the site when it was submitted to the directory to decide whether a site matches the searcher's needs. For both there is little or no selection in terms of quality of information, although engines and directories do try to impose rules about decency and content. Popular search engines in the UK include:

google.co.uk
aol.co.uk
msn.co.uk
lycos.co.uk
hotbot.co.uk
overture.com
ask.co.uk
espotting.com
looksmart.co.uk

alltheweb.com
uk.altavista.com

The two biggest directories are:

yahoo.com
dmoz.org

Portals

Portals are doorways to the internet that provide links to useful sites, news and other services, and may also provide search engine services (such as msn.co.uk). Many portals charge for putting their clients' sites high up in your list of search results. The quality of the websites listed depends on the selection criteria used in compiling the portal, although portals focused on a specific group, such as medical information portals, may have more rigorous inclusion criteria than other searchable websites. Examples of medical portals can be found at:

nhsdirect.nhs.uk
patient.co.uk

Links to many British medical charities will be found at the Association of Medical Research Charities (www.amrc.org.uk) and Charity Choice (www.charitychoice. co.uk).

Search phrases

Be specific when entering a search phrase. Searching for information on 'cancer' could give astrological information as well as medical: 'lung cancer' would be a better choice. Either use the engine's advanced search feature and ask for the exact phrase, or put the phrase in quotes – 'lung cancer' – as this will link the words. Adding 'uk' to your search phrase will bring up mainly British websites, so a good search would be 'lung cancer' uk (don't include uk within the quotes).

Always remember that the internet is international and unregulated. Although it holds a wealth of invaluable information, individual websites may be biased, out of date or just plain wrong. Family Doctor Publications accepts no responsibility for the content of links published in their series.

Index